ELECTROPHOTONIC

APPLICATIONS

IN MEDICINE

GDV

BIOELECTROGRAPHY

RESEARCH

Dr. Ekaterina Yakovleva

Dr. Konstantin Korotkov

1

Electrophotonic Applications in Medicine.
GDV Bioelectrography research.

Dr. Ekaterina Yakovleva and Dr. Konstantin Korotkov

This book is a survey of papers dedicated to Electrophotonic Imaging (EPI) GDV Bioelectrography applications in Medicine and Psychology from 2000 to 2012. The most of cited works are presented in proceedings of different conferences, but a lot are published in per-review journals. It is clear that Electrophotonic technique has high potential in analyzing Human Energy Field for health and wellbeing and monitoring the reaction of people to different influences and treatments.

Dr. Ekaterina Yakovleva, M.D., Ph.D., Professor of the Russian National Research Medical University named after N.I. Pirogov, Moscow, Russia, and author of many papers published in per-review journals. From 1999 develops applications of Electtrophotonic Analysis in medicine. She has published 35 papers and a monography on this topic in Russian journals.

Dr. Konstantin Korotkov, Ph.D., Professor of Computer Science and Biophysics at Saint-Petersburg Federal Research University of Informational Technologies, Mechanics and Optics. Deputy Director of Saint-Petersburg Federal Research Institute of Physical Culture and Sport. He has published over 200 papers in leading journals on physics and biology, and he holds 17 patents on biophysics inventions.

ISBN 978-1481932981

Contents

Books by Dr Konstantin Korotkov

Korotkov K. Light After Life. Backbone publishing, NY. 1998. 190 p.

Korotkov K. Aura and Consciousness – New Stage of Scientific Understanding. St.Petersburg, Russian Ministry of Culture. 1998. 270 p. ISBN 5-8334-0330-8.

Korotkov K. Human Energy Field: study with GDV bioelectrography. Backbone publishing, NY. 2002. 360 p.

Measuring Energy Fields: State of the Art. GDV Bioelectrography series. Korotkov K. (Ed.). Backbone Publishing Co. Fair Lawn, USA, 2004. 270 p.

Korotkov K. Spiral Traverse. St. Petersburg, 2006.

Korotkov K. Champs D'Energie Humaine. Resurgence Collection. Belgique. 2005

Korotkov K., Carlos Mejia Osorio. La Bioelectrografia. Baranquilla. Colombia. 2005.

Korotkov. K. Geheimnisse des lebendigen Leuchtens. Herstellung Leipzig, Germany, 2006, 142 p.

Korotkov K.G. Les Principles De L'Analyse GDV. Marco Pietteur, Editeur, Belgue, 2009

Korotkov K.G. Energy fields Electrophotonic analysis in humans and nature. 2012. 240 p. e-book: Amazon.com

Science Confirms Reconnective Healing: Frontier Science Experiments. Authored by Dr. Konstantin Korotkov. 2012. 152 p. Amazon.com Publishing.

Korotkov K.G. The Energy of Consciousness. 2012. 220 p. Amazon.com Publishing.

Abbreviations

AP   - arterial pressure
BA   - Bronchial Asthma
EPI   - Electrophotonic Imaging
GDV   - Gas Discharge Visualization
GDI   - Gas Discharge Image
S   - GDI background area
I   - Averaged Intensity
E   - Energy of light in Jouls $E = S * I * 0.00002$
JgS   - Integral area coefficient
EC   - Emission coefficient
FC   - Form coefficient
FrC   - Fractality coefficient
FS   - Functional systems

INTRODUCTION

Pages of History

Although claims for the existence of energy fields have been widely accepted in various Eastern medical practices for many centuries, claims concerning the reality of human energy fields were rejected by Western scientists because they considered that objective evidence for their existence was not available. This situation began to change somewhat during the latter part of the nineteenth century when photographs were made of the electrical discharges from animate and inanimate objects. This was based on the effect discovered in 1777 by German physicist and philosopher George Lichtenberg. He has found that if any object be placed in strong electrical field one can see glow around the object. Lichtenberg was able to print images on a plate covered with coal dust and it became known in physics as "Lichtenberg' figures". The term "electrography" was coined to describe these images explored by the Czech physicist Navratil in 1888. In essence, a high intensity electric field is created around an object which produces a gas discharge. Since this discharge is accompanied by photon emission it can be photographed.

The interest in photographing electrical fluorescence arose all over the world after the experiments of Nicola Tesla. He had developed special coils named after him and demonstrated that high voltage may be absolutely safe (of course, if you know how to use it). A significant contribution to the study of electrography images was made by a talented Byelorussian scientist Jacob Narkevich-Yodko in the end of the Nineteenth century. He was an independent landowner and spent most of his time on his estate above the river Neman. There he actively experimented with electricity, applying it in agriculture and medicine. A straight parallel with modern medicine can be drawn from the description of experiments on the stimulation of plants with electrical current, on electrotherapy, and magnetism by J. Narkevich-Yodko. In the end of the Nineteenth century, when the principles of electricity were only emerging, when the main source of light was a kerosene lamp, the searching investigators were trying to apply electricity to the most different areas of life. They were as if naming the chapters of a new book, but had not enough power to write the contents. Therefore, we find the sources of one or another modern scientific direction in the works of the enthusiasts of the Nineteenth century.

J. Narkevich-Yodko developed his own original technique for making electrophotographs. He made more than 1500 photographs of fingers of different people, plant leaves, grain, and in the 1890's this research attracted attention in the scientific community. In 1892 J. Narkevich-Yodko presented for the professors of St. Petersburg Institute of Experimental Medicine, after which he was appointed a "Member-Employee of this Institute" by the order of the Institute patron, the Prince of Oldenburg. The results of Narkevich-Yodko created such an impression upon the scientific community that in 1893 a conference on electrography and electrophysiology was organized in St. Petersburg University. In the same year Narkevich-Yodko visited the scientific centers of Europe: Berlin, Vienna, Paris, Prague, Florence and gave lectures there. His experiments on electrography were acknowledged as important and envisaging further development everywhere. Narkevich Yodko received medals at several exhibitions, and at the Congress in France in 1900 he was nominated a professor of electrography and magnetism.

J. Narkevich-Yodko combined scientific work with public activity. He organized a health center on his estate and received people from very different social circles: from grandees to plain people, and cured many different diseases with the help of the newest for those days, methods. But with the death of J. Narkevich-Yodko the contemporaries forgot his works. He made an interesting discovery, but could not overcome the barrier which had always been in the road of wide introduction. The general social situation in Russia played a role in the life of Narkevich-Yodko. Evil social winds were blowing, which turned into a hurricane having destroyed the leisurely way of life of the Nineteenth century and changed the beautiful estates above the Neman and Volga rivers into cold abandoned ruins. «No prophet is accepted in his own country», especially when this prophet thinks in a non-standard way and doesn't fall into the usual pattern. But can a Prophet live a normal life?

At practically the same time, on the other side of the globe in Brazil, very similar experiments were performed by a Catholic monk, padre Landell de Morua. This was a funny little man with a long nose, disappointed in the vanity of the worldly life – and bound to devote himself to serving God. A monk's life left a lot of free time, after reading prayers and performing rituals. Some of the monks went in for gardening and sometimes, as Gregor Mendel, invented new laws of nature; somebody else researched ancient civilizations, which were all over the place in South America; but padre de Morua started inventing. He invented the technique of photoregistration of electrical glow and started giving lectures and writing to social leaders in order to attract attention to his offspring. But Brazil is not the USA. In Brazil everybody enjoys life, dances, prepares for the carnival for half a year and continuously sorts out emotional relationships. Have you watched Brazilian soap operas? They live like that in reality. Well, probably, not so many intrigues. It is too hot there in summer to trouble oneself with much effort. I had a chance to be in Brazil at conferences, I will tell later about that, and every time it was a Holiday with a plenty of food, wine, songs, and dances. Therefore, it is no wonder that the invention of padre de Morua produced much rapt attention, congratulations, banquets, but was not widespread. Then the little big-nose priest invented the radio (practically simultaneously with Popov and Markoni), but again he was unable to draw in large crowds. Even the military. Generals admired, realized the importance and perspectives of the wireless communication, promised to call the colonel the next day and assign resources, but in an hour left for a night's banquet and forgot about everything.

In 1939, Semyon Kirlian, a Russian electrician, rediscovered this phenomenon and he and his wife Valentina began exploring the possible significance of the colored "auras" or coronas that he found surrounding the various objects that he photographed with his technique (Kirlian and Kirlian, 1961). And, when the images started to be registered and not just admired, it was found that the picture of fingertips' glow depended of the subject. Someone felt nervous or, on the contrary, fell into a meditative trance, and the photo of glow changed its form. Due to these effects Kirlian photography subsequently became a topic of wide interest to European and American investigators.One of the most extensive American investigations was carried out at the UCLA Center for the Health Sciences. T. Moss and K. Johnson (1973) indicated that they had taken more than 10,000 'modified' Kirlian photographs, chiefly of the human fingertip, leaves, and metal objects. More than 500 hundred persons and more than 1,000 leaves were photographed. They found that a subject's energy field was affected by ingesting alcohol, performing yogic breathing, undergoing hypnosis, or experiencing emotional states. After carrying out several careful experiments, the investigators were able to conclude that the electrophotographs were not due to skin resistance, nor to the state of the peripheral vascular system.

In an interesting series of experiments, the researchers found intriguing patterns of interpersonal influence on the photographs. The corona usually differed when the experimenter and subject were of different genders as opposed to when they were of the same gender, and a strict authority figure, such as an elderly experimenter, usually produced a much smaller corona than an informal friendly assistant. In research with four "healers", the healers' coronas were found to be much larger and brighter before the healing session than during or after healing. In contrast, the patients' coronas increased sharply over their pre-healing states, as if an actual transfer of energy were occurring between the healer and her patient. Dramatic differences in the corona were found before and after acupuncture treatment. The brightness and clarity of the corona were particularly noticeable if the needles were inserted at points known to be related to a patient's specific physical complaints.

Another American researcher, L.W. Konikiewicz (1979), under careful laboratory conditions using double-blind studies, correctly identified cystic fibrosis patients and carriers of the gene with a high order of accuracy. He also found that the day of the menstrual cycle influenced variations in the brightness of the energy field and that the day of ovulation could be detected. The patterns were different for subjects taking an oral contraceptive. In a later revised edition of his book, co-authored with L.C. Griff (1984), results were reported about their success in detecting cancer and other abnormal physiological conditions.

Scientific acceptance of Kirlian photography has been rather limited, however, because the type of equipment used in earlier years varied quite markedly from investigator to investigator and there was a wide range of parameters that needed to be controlled for the successful operation of the method. A multi-disciplinary team, headed for several years by William Eidson at Drexel University in Philadelphia, concluded it was possible to image electrical parameters of a specimen in real time, making it a possible field- mapping tool for energy fields. This work was summarized in an article in the prestigious journal *Science* (Pehek et al. 1976).

In the technological area, an organization to help standardize equipment output parameters, research methods, data presentation standards etc. called the International Union of Medical and Applied Bio-Electrography was formed in 1987. Professor Korotkov was elected as a President of the Union in 2000 at the World Congress in Brazil and then re-elected in 2006. At the present time, investigators in 68 countries are currently pursuing a variety of studies with the latest Electrography Imaging technology that will be described in the next sections. International conferences to present the latest findings have been held for the last 17 years in St. Petersburg, Russia.

Part I. PRINCIPLES OF ELECTROPHOTONIC ANALYSIS

How Does Electrophotonic/GDV Technique Assess a Body?

*Williams B., Korotkov K.

*University of Kansas and University of Integrative Medicine, USA,
berneyw@ku.edu

The Electrophotonic Imaging – EPI Technique, based on Gas Discharge Visualization process is well characterized in the physical processes by which it captures and analyzes data. This paper explores candidate mechanisms in physiology and biophysics through which EPI data from biological subjects can reflect the state of health in human beings. Increasing numbers of clinical studies show that particular details in EPI data correlate with conditions that can be characterized using standard medical diagnostics, as well as correlating with assessment methods used in a wide range of complementary medicine.

Previous discussions [K Korotkov, B. Williams and L. A. Wisneski, 2004] have proposed that EPI assessment methods can be understood using quantum biophysical models of entropy and information flows as follows: A main reservoir of free energy in biological processes is electron-excited states of complex molecular systems. This quantum model supports an argument that EPI techniques provide indirect judgment about the level of energy resources at the molecular level in structure-protein complexes. Collections of delocalized excited π-electrons in protein macromolecules provide an energy reservoir for physiological processes. Delocalization means that the collection of π- electrons is distributed in a certain way over the entire structure of a molecular complex. This enables the π-electrons not only to migrate within the limits of their own molecule, but also to transfer from one molecule to another, if the molecules are structurally united into ensembles. The most important mission of π-electrons in biological processes derives not only from their delocalization, but also from the peculiarities of their energy

11

status. The difference between the energies of the main and the excited state is much smaller for π-electrons than for σ-electrons (local electrons). The transformation of electron energy in biostructures is connected not only with transfer of electrons, but also with the migration of electronic excitation energy, which does not include electron detachment from a donor's molecule. Inductive-resonance, exchange-resonance, and excitonic mechanisms for transfer of electronic excitation turn out to be the most important for biological systems. These processes are significant when we consider energy transfers in molecular complexes, which aren't, as a rule, followed by a transfer of charge.

Specific structural-protein complexes within the mass of the skin provide channels of heightened electron conductivity, measurable at acupuncture points on the skin surface. Stimulated impulse emissions from the skin are also developed mainly by transport of delocalized π-electrons. Stimulated by high voltage impulses, optical emissions amplified in gaseous discharge, are registered by optical sensors in the EPI technique. Television capture of the time dynamics of this glow from the skin, with a scale of some millimeters in diameter, and frame-by-frame comparison of these pictures of fluorescence during each voltage impulse show that the emission centers appear approximately from the same skin points. Ion-depolarization processes in the tissue have no time to develop within the short periods of EPI stimulation of 10 nsec, therefore the current may be resulting from the transport of electrons within structural complexes of skin or other biological tissue under investigation, included in the chain of impulse electrical current flow. Biological tissues are assumed to be divided into dielectrics and conductors (primarily biological conducting liquids). In order to unite the effects of stimulated electron emission, it is necessary to consider electron transport mechanisms along non-conducting structures. Most attention in this sphere has been focused on concepts of electron tunnel transport between separate protein molecules-carriers, separated from one another by energy barriers. The processes of electron tunnel transport are experimentally well studied and modeled by the example of transferring electrons along the protein chain. The tunnel mechanism provides the initial act of electron transfer between donor-acceptor groups in the protein, each being within $0.5 - 1.0$ nm distance from one another. There are also many examples, however, where the electron is transferred within the protein for much longer distances. It is thus essential that the transfer can take place not only within the limits of one protein molecule, but may also involve the interaction of different protein structures. The characteristic time of electron transfer ranges between 10-11 and 10-6 sec, which corresponds to the development time for a single emission act in the EPI technique.

Building on this prior discussion, the present paper explores further possible mechanisms for communication of internal physiological states to the skin surface, where stimulated emissions provide EPI information. New ideas about the role of biophotonic resonance processes for maintaining coordinated metabolic action, [1] and the role of water and reactive oxygen species (ROS) in providing information flow, energy reservoirs and energy pumping, [2,3] all emphasize the potential for extended models of physiological communication and control. Recent biophysical research reveals a wide range of properties that enable the body to use sound, light, electricity, magnetic fields, heat, elasticity, torsion and other forms of vibration as signals for integrating and coordinating diverse physiological activities [4].

James Oschman has explored concepts of communication and coordination in physiological processes, connecting all levels of physical organization through what he calls a "Living Matrix," reaching from processes in the nuclei of cells through the intracellular dynamics mediated by the cellular cytoskeleton and communicating through the cell membranes to connective tissues ramifying throughout the body. Key innovations have been the recognition of processes involved with the intracellular cytoskeleton and the connective tissues in physiology at extra-cellular levels. Historically biochemistry developed along lines focused on chemical processes of molecular formation, emphasizing the energy economy of reduction/oxidation reactions, with enzyme catalysis and hormone regulation as main sources of coordination and modulation. Newly developing perspectives are going beyond these processes, examining electronic semi-conduction and quantum electronic processes involving resonant states of complex molecular systems. Enzyme catalysis is now being explored as a process regulated by quantum tunneling [5] and Luca Turin has proposed a model in which the olfactory sense identifies molecules by detecting interior molecular bonding structures using electron tunneling "spectroscopy." [6] Hameroff was one of the first to propose information processing along the microtubules in cells using quantum coherence processes.[7]

A striking aspect of EPI data is the strong correlation with signal and energy flows associated with the acupuncture meridians. Various models have been explored for the mechanisms of acupuncture. Strong evidence exists for the reality and physiological character of acupuncture processes. Histological studies have identified unique tissue arrangements at

13

acupuncture points, involving a lymphatic trunk entwined by an arteriol and an associated small vein. The lymph and blood vessels are surrounded by networks of unmylenated cholenergic autonomic nerves. The entire complex at each acupuncture point is embedded in a column of loosely arranged connective tissue, enclosed in a boundary of more densely packed connective tissue. The interaction of these anatomical processes make acupuncture points a network of nodes interfacing between the body's matrix of connective tissues and the major circulatory and neural regulatory systems.[8,9,10] And new evidence is gathering for signal and energy flows along the "Living Matrix" of the connective tissues and cellular cytoskeleton. Strong evidence previously was seen for ion flow along lamina in tissue as part of the acupuncture processes. Evidence has recently also been found for ultra-high speed signal flow associated with acupuncture systems an order of magnitude faster than neurological signals.[11]

Mae-Wan Ho proposes a multilayed physiological energy and information system: "The extracellular, intracellular, and nuclear matrices together constitute a noiseless excitable electronic continuum for rapid intercommunication and energy flow permeating the entire organism, enabling it to function as a coherent and sentient whole."[12] Her insights focus on coordination and communication processes across multiple levels of physiology, with the tissues of the entire organism acting as a liquid crystal continuum, passing information and energy up and down within systems and subsystems, coordinated throughout the Living Matrix.[13] Testing with the EPI perturbs an organism with stimulating voltage pulses, creating miniature displacements of the holistic regulatory system. Similar to holographic processes, this transaction with a small part reveals the responsiveness of the whole. Any maladjusted organ system shows a disordered sector in the corona discharge at the associated fingertip. Analysis in the frequency domains of EPI data could reveal subtle multi-layered systemic resonance. The potential for such frequency domain analysis has been seen in an assessment of EPI data that correctly identified the driving frequency profile in an acoustic binaural beat entrainment stimulus during a single subject session at the Monroe Institute in Virginia.

References

[1] F. A. Popp, "Some Remarks on Biological Consequence of a Coherent Biophoton Field," in F. A. Popp, K. H. Li and Q. Gu, editors, Recent Advances in Biophoton Research and its Applications," Singapore/ River Edge, NJ/London, 1992, pp. 357-373

[2] V. Voeikov, "Mitogenetic radiation, biophotons, and non-linear oxidative processes in aqueous media," in Integrative Biophysics, Biphotonics, F. A. Popp, L. Beloussov, editors, Kluwer Academic Publishers, Dordrecht/Bosont/London, 2003 pp. 331-360.

[3] V. L. Voeikov, "Processes Involving Reactive Oxygen Species are the Major Source of Structured energy for Organismal Biophotonic Field Pumping," in L. Beloussov, F-A. Popp, V. Voeikov, and R. Van Wijk, editors, Biophotonics and Coherent Systems, Proceedings of the 2nd Alexander Gurwitsch Conference and Additional Contributions, Moscow University Press, Moscow, 2000.

[4] J. Oschman, Energy Medicine in Therapeutics and Human Performance, Butterworth Heinemann, 2003.

[5] A. Kohen and J. P. Klinman, "Protein Flexibility Correlates with Degree of Hydrogen Tunneling in Thermophilic and Mesophilic Alcohol Dehydrogenases," J. of the American Chemical Society, 2000, V 122, pp. 10738-10739.

[6] L. Turin, "Structure-odor relations: a modern perspective," in R. L. Doty, editor, Handbook of Olfaction and Gustation 2nd ed. Marcel Dekker, New York, NY, 2003.

[7] S. R. Hameroff,"Coherence in the cytoskeleton: Implication for biological information processing," in H. Frohlich H., editor, Biological Coherence and Response to External Stimuli, Springer-Verlag, Berlin, 1988, pp. 242-263.

[8] O. Auziech, Etude Histologique des Points Cutane de Moindre Resistance Electrique et Analyse de Leurs Implications Possibles Dans la Mise en Jeu des Mecanismes Acupuncturaux, These de Medecine, Montpellier, 1984.

[9] C. Vallette and J. -E. -H. Niboyet, Gynecologie-Obstetrique: Therapeutique par Acupuncture, MEDSI (Medecine et Sciences International), Paris, 1981

[10] R. Senelar, Caracteristiques morphologiques des points chinois, in J. -E, -H. Niboyet, editor, Nouveau Traite d'Acupuncture, Maisonneuve, Moulins-les-Metz, 1979, pp. 247-277.

[11] Z. H. Cho, S. C. Chung, J. P. Jones, J. B. Park, H. J. Park, H. J. Lee, E. K. Wong and R. I Min, "New findings of the correlation between acupoints and corresponding brain cortices using functional MR," Proceedings of the National Academy of Sciences of the USA, V 95 N 5, 1998, pp. 2670-2673.

[12] M. W. Ho, "Quantum coherence and conscious experience," Kybernetics, 1997, V 26, pp. 265-276.

[13] M. W. Ho, The Rainbow and the Worm: The Physics of Organisms, 2nd ed, World Scientific, Singapore, 1998.

Basic rules of EPI analysis

In order to correctly analyze the physiological state, i.e. the level of energy of the organs and the systems (or in other words, the level of autonomic regulation, in accordance with the adaptation levels) it is necessary to take the following steps:

Different EPI programs reflect different aspects of a person's energy status. EPI-grams must be processed in all programs and it is advisable to print out the following:

- EPI-grams of all fingers without filter;
- EPI-grams of all fingers with filter;
- EPI diagrams;
- All EPI EF (Energy Field) projections.

When classifying EPI data by adaptation level, we look at the following factors:

- Specific features on EPI-grams wF and F;
- Distribution of EPI diagrams wF and F.

The **H homeostasis zone** is characterized as follows:

- EPI wF have a small number of defects;
- EPI F have no defects;
- Both Diagrams lie in the optimal zone;
- The level of activation $0 < A \leq 5$;
- Diagram variance < 0.5.

The **HS homeostasis zone** is characterized as follows:

- EPI wF have defects;
- EPI F do not have substantial defects, but are more heterogeneous than in H zone.
- Diagram without filter lie totally or partially in the energy deficit zone;

16

- Diagram with filter may have energy deficit zones;
- R-L imbalance;
- Level of activation $2.5 \leq A \leq 10$;
- Diagram variance > 0.5;

In H and HS homeostasis zones, we apply sector analysis.

The **P homeostasis zone** is characterized as follows:

- EPI wF have a specific 'partial-continuous' appearance or are distinguished by a large number of defects on all fingers;
- EPI F have a specific 'cloudy' structure in a number of sectors. The more sectors there are with this structure, the worse the condition.
- EPI F have a large number of defects and homogeneity.
- Diagrams lie in the upper limit of the optimal zone or beyond it.
- The level of activation does not provide useful information.

The **ASC homeostasis zone** is characterized as follows:

- EPI wF have specific defects in the form of individual blotches, branches or double rings.
- EPI F can have the same appearance as is characteristic of H and P homeostasis zones, while also being distinguished by a large quantity of 'blanks-holes'.
- Diagrams wF have the typical 'starry' appearance.
- The sectorial diagnosis in P and ASC homeostasis zones can be applied with greater accuracy.
- A high level of 'background' noise is typical of increased physiological activity in the body's systems, linked to the high level of activation.
- During analysis, the age and gender of the patient should be taken into account; these factors are included in the evaluations by EPI programs.

17

Fingers of left hand

Fingers of right hand

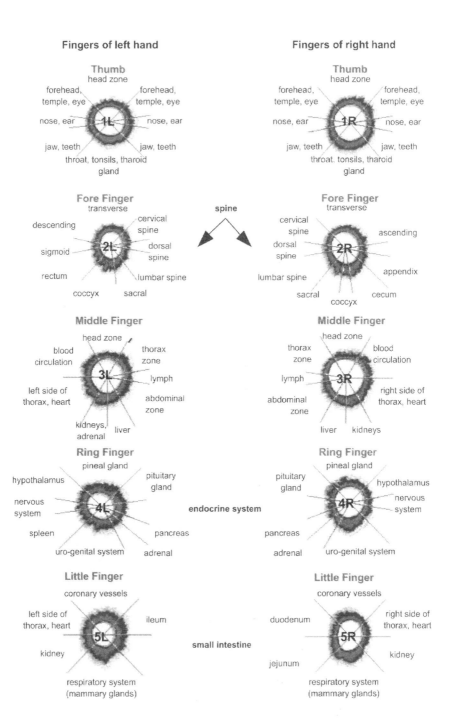

Thumb
head zone
forehead, temple, eye — forehead, temple, eye
nose, ear — 1L — nose, ear
jaw, teeth — jaw, teeth
throat, tonsils, tharoid gland

Thumb
head zone
forehead, temple, eye — forehead, temple, eye
nose, ear — 1R — nose, ear
jaw, teeth — jaw, teeth
throat, tonsils, tharoid gland

Fore Finger
transverse
descending — cervical spine
2L — dorsal spine
sigmoid
rectum — lumbar spine
coccyx — sacral

spine

Fore Finger
transverse
cervical spine — ascending
dorsal spine — 2R
lumbar spine — appendix
sacral — cecum
coccyx

Middle Finger
head zone
blood circulation — thorax zone
3L — lymph
left side of thorax, heart — abdominal zone
kidneys, adrenal — liver

Middle Finger
head zone
thorax zone — blood circulation
lymph — 3R
abdominal zone — right side of thorax, heart
liver — kidneys

Ring Finger
pineal gland
hypothalamus — pituitary gland
nervous system — 4L
spleen — pancreas
uro-genital system — adrenal

endocrine system

Ring Finger
pineal gland
pituitary gland — hypothalamus
4R — nervous system
pancreas
adrenal — uro-genital system

Little Finger
coronary vessels
left side of thorax, heart — ileum
5L
kidney
respiratory system (mammary glands)

small intestine

Little Finger
coronary vessels
duodenum — right side of thorax, heart
5R
jejunum — kidney
respiratory system (mammary glands)

18

With appropriate calibration, diagrams can give very important information. We pay attention not only to the energy of particular systems and organs, but also to the interrelation between wF and F curves. Additionally, differences between right and left diagrams may be an indication of troublesome information.

The types of EPI-grams reviewed in the book *Human Energy Field: Study with GDV-bioelectrography,* are inherent to all levels of activation and are a compound element of the means of interpretation carried out in this method. Those EPI-grams can be used during specification, however, so as not to confuse perceptions, we have left out that complicated text in this discussion.

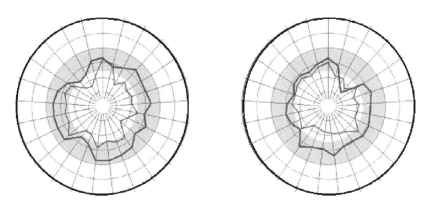

GDV Diagram

Following the specified practice, the EPI method makes it possible to carry out a reasonably accurate analysis of the physical and psychological state of the patient. To a large extent, the accuracy of the analysis depends on the depth of understanding of systemic principles of how the body works, and whether it is perceived as a unified, holistic, indivisible system. In order to work out such an approach, some knowledge of the principles of Traditional Chinese Medicine (TCM) is very helpful. They are based on the idea of the circulation of energy, and these ideas are fully reflected in the practice of EPI bioelectrography. We gauge the movement of energy through systems and organs, and in many examples we can see the direct reflection of the principles of TCM.

In addition, knowledge of these principles facilitates the development of clinical intuition, and, by placing reasonable trust in one's

19

own 'inner voice,' it is possible to make an accurate and in many cases unexpected analysis based on EPI data. Many doctors who have used EPI over many years have indicated similar experiences.

Trust the information provided by the EPI data without concerning yourself with the outward appearance of the patient. In the case of systemic illnesses, appearance is deceptive. EPI pictures give authentic information on the person's energy state.

A totally intuitive path of analysis was developed by M. Shaduri based on the intuitive identification of images of organs in EPI images. This path is based on intuitive guesswork, and EPI images play the same role as Tarot cards - by giving information to those with a gift – but they are not an objective means of analysis.

Specially designed programs allow for easy calculation of GDV-gram parameters generated in the routine process of patient investigation.

To properly characterize the GDV-gram the following indices are used: **GDI background area, averaged Intensity, Energy, normalized area, integral area coefficient, emission coefficient, form coefficient, fractality coefficient** along with dispersions of all mentioned parameters.

GDI background area (S) is an absolute value and is measured in pixels.

Averaged Intensity (I) is evaluation of light intensity averaged on the area of the image.

Energy (E) of light in Jouls is calculated from the experiments as

$$E = S * I * 0.00002$$

Normalized area is the ratio of GDI area to the area of the inner oval - a non-informative part of the image and is obtained as a result of placing the finger onto a GDV camera electrode; as essentially a background or baseline value, it is reported in relative units.

Integral area coefficient (JgS) is a relative value and shows the extent to which the GDV-gram area of the examined patient deviates to one or the other side from an ideal model. Naturally, this parameter can have a positive or negative value; moreover, in the case where it is equal to zero, it indicates that the test image and the area of the ideal model is the same.

Emission coefficient (EC) characterizes the power of small fragments deleted from the GDV-gram and is measured in pixels.

Form coefficient (FC) is calculated according to the formula: $FC = L*2/S$, where L is the length of the GDI external contour and S is the GDI background area.

Fractality coefficient (FrC) is calculated according to the algorithm of Mandelbro as a ratio of the lengths of GDI parameters, provided that the GDI is registered several times and averaged. Form and fractality coefficients show the degree of irregularity of the GDV-gram external contour.

In the process of research, separate measurements to obtain the values of these indices for each finger, average values of the indices for fingers of both hands, and particularly individual assessment for the right vs. the left hands is obtained.

For evaluation of the functional state of particular functional systems (FS) and organs, these parameters are calculated in the sectors of FS's projecting zones as introduced by P. Mandel [1986] and interpreted by K. Korotkov [1998]. Evaluation of functional states for different FS is done by estimating the heterogeneity of the GDV-gram in particular sectors, the degree of aggressive signs intensity on the right and left hands for different interconnected sectors, as well as for individual fingers. Based upon this evaluation and in consideration of the clinical picture of the disease, analysis is made and conclusions drawn.

It is noteworthy that GDV-gram parameters which fall within the zone of relative health as characterized by the average range determined for practically healthy people, do not exclude the presence of chronic diseases to which a patient may have good compensatory capabilities. Reductions in bioenergetic activities of the patient, e.g. in the phase of resolution of an exacerbation of chronic diseases during rehabilitation (such as resolving asthmatic crisis) might be the basis for prescribing methods of therapy. This might include promoting and activating energy homeokinesis and renewal of normal interaction of all the FS of the organism.

Clinical observations with GDV-bioelectrography when people have vegetative instability results in considerable asymmetry of parameters' values for the left and right hands (i.e. lateralization); this data can infer evidence of a decreased adaptation reserve of an individual's energy homeokinesis, and perhaps be viewed as predictive. If the 'weak zones' with the modified values of parameters in the presence of clinical symptoms and pathology are correlated with the corresponding FS, the patient could be assessed and managed for these dysfunctions and energetic imbalances through a composite program including both conventional and complementary modalities. GDV-bioelectrography could help assess the monitoring for efficacy and re-establishment of a normalized auric field such as found in practically healthy people.

Special attention to the role of vegetative nervous system in the developing of big variety of different disorders and their representations on bio-electrograms was poited out by Professors of Russian Medical Academy of Post-Graduate Education Drozdov D.A. and Shatsillo O.I. [2005]. They wrote: "The decisive role in the formation of the prerequisites for the appearance and development of the diseases belongs to the mechanisms of adaptation to various factors of external and internal environment, controlled by the vegetative part of the central nervous system, and to the extent of the compensation of the disturbed functions. This role of the vegetative nervous system is ensured by the anatomic-functional hierarchy of its structural components represented by the central and peripheral sections. The GDV-bioelectrography technique proved to be the most informative and convenient diagnostics method in application. It is especially valuable for the objectivization of the vegetative disorders. Analysis of the GDV-grams taken without filter displayed optical effects (taking into account the complex vegetative influences on the skin) which result in the glow area decrease, fractality increase and the fragmentation of the obtained image up to the complete disappearance of the glow. The filter that is used for the registration of the BEO-grams of fingers cuts off the information related to the vegetative influences on the skin (both sympathetic and parasympathetic). The GDV-grams taken with filter display optical effects related to the operation of the morphological structures of the organism which generates bioelectricity. And the glow area displays the integral energy resource of the organism – an integral parameter of the electromagnetic field of the organism".

Gender and age dependence

In several papers was demonstrated that there are significant statistical difference in GDV parameters between genders. As a whole energy parameters for women are higher compared with men.

In a group of people statistical distribution of the GDV parameters without filter follows log-normal distribution, typical for biological subjects. In a group of middle-aged apparently healthy people (31-52 years old) distribution has a tail in lower values, while in a group of yang people (18-21 yers old) the tail goes to the higher values. That means that in middle-aged group there are some people with very low energy, while in a yang group there are several people with very high energy.

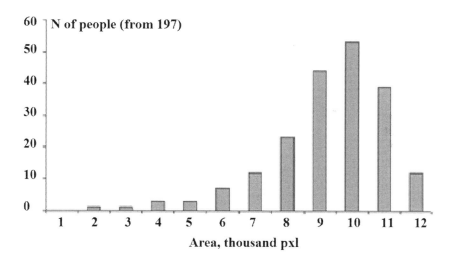

Fig. Statistical distribution of the GDV Area parameter without filter for a group of middle-aged people.

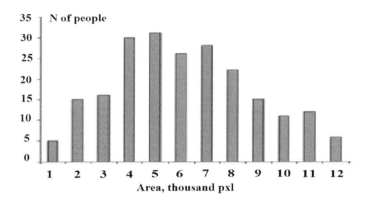

Fig. Statistical distribution of the GDV Area parameter without filter for a group of yang people.

Statistical distribution of the GDV Area with filter is more close to normal distribution.

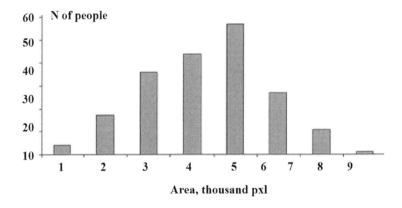

Fig. Statistical distribution of the GDV Area parameter with filter for a group of middle-aged people.

Detailed discussion of age and gender difference for the whole set of EPI indexes is presented in the paper [Ciesielska-Wrobel et al 2010] based on the study of population of 126 persons (81 men and 45 women).

From this we have to conclude that in quantitative analysis data for women and men as well as for different age groups should be evaluated differently.

Reproducibility

This topic was first addressed in the paper of [Russo M et al 2001]. By quantitative analysis they demonstrated that reproducibility of GDV data for most people is more than 90% but we need to take into account physiological cycles and the influence of emotions, alcohol, medications and quality of sleep.

By performing daily monitoring the **reproducibility of GDV parameters' values** was investigated for 38 practically healthy people and in 30 bronchial asthma (BA) patients [Alexandrova, 2001]. 38 healthy people and 20 asthmatic patients with a 10-minute interval, 20 practically healthy and 20 asthmatic patients with a day interval and 22 sick people within a day: at 9 a.m., 1, 5, 9 p.m. and 9 a.m. next day. For the healthy people the values of amplitudes of the GDV-gram parameters' fluctuations, daily average and average 10-minute, amounted to 4.1 and 6.6%, for BA patients - respectively - 8.6 and 7.7% .

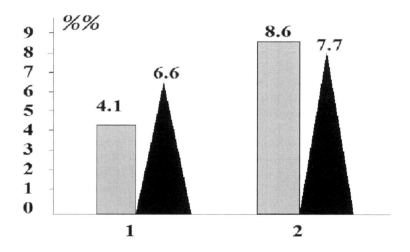

Fig. Fluctuation of GDV parameters for healthy people (rectangles) and bronchial asthma patients averaged daily (1) and in 10-minutes (2).

A group of individuals (10% of all examined, BA and healthy people) was identified in which the variability of the GDV-gram parameters registered considerably higher - up to 18% over the daily average value. So we may accept that reproducibility of GDV indexes for practically healthy, mentally stable people should be better than 90% and all variations exceeding this level may be considered as significant. This is important when we evaluate the effect of some influence or treatment.

The influence of atmospheric conditions to a group of people was studied by [Dunlop 2004]. Room temperature (ranged from 71 to 84 degrees) and barometric pressure (ranged from 29 to 31 degrees) were negatively correlated with the fourth finger entropy value. Increases in room temperature and a rise in room barometric pressure had a negative effect on the endocrine energy condition. In contrast, GDV fourth finger entropy value measures were positively correlated with humidity (ranged from 61% to 83%): as the percentage of humidity rose, the endocrine entropy condition rose. **Entropy** values increased in reaction to the effects of higher humidity on the individual. Entropy reflects the level of non-uniformity of the GDV image, in other words, the level of stability of the Energy Field. After [Gibson 2004] we may attribute it to the texture of an image: lower entropy is correlated with firm and fine texture, while high entropy is characteristic of coarse, porous, broken contour of an image.

Recommended procedures

1. Calibrate the EPI device and EPI programs at least four times a year, or if conditions change, e.g. moving the camera to another site, change of computer, severe change in atmospheric conditions. Calibration must also be performed if 'unusual' results are obtained.

2. Check the capture parameters in the EPI Camera (in accordance with the device instructions) and the processing parameters in programs. **Changing the processing parameters leads to distorted results.**

3. Take EPI images of the patient at least 2 hours after the consumption of a large quantity of food, without alcohol or strong medicines. **Some medicines (in particular, hormones or anti-depressants) will have an effect on the nature of the energy. It is advisable to empty the bladder and bowels before image capturing begins.**

4. The examination of the patients may be conducted during all the day, but preferably before any medical diagnostic procedures and the intake of drugs, at least two hours after the latest intake of food and smoking, and at least 24 hours after the latest intake of alcohol. The intake of certain drugs influences the psychophysiological state.

5. The fingers must not be washed or wiped with alcohol before the registration. If the hands are very dirty, wash and wait a further 15 minutes.

6. **In the case of sweaty hands** (excessive perspiration), wipe each finger individually and then take EPI images.

7. Before taking EPI images it is advisable to allow the patient to relax for 15 minutes, drink water (but not tea or coffee) and sit in pleasant surroundings with relaxing music.

8. Some people, particularly children and the young, may demonstrate a 'medical reaction' which manifests itself as a stress reaction on the measurement process.

9. **Before each measurement, the optic lens of the EPI device must be wiped clean.**

10. If unusual EPI-grams are obtained, repeat the measurement of the patient and be sure that the results are precise.

11. It is necessary to use a new filter for taking EPI images of ten fingers of each patient. Ensure that the filter is accurately stored, straightened out and does not become crushed during the measurements.

12. Repeated image capturing may lead to varying results. Decreased

of the EPI-gram indicats deregulation of adaptation levels. In such cases, it is necessary to carry out a series of repeated measurements and draw conclusions accordingly. Each series of EPI images must be taken both with and without filter.

13. Psychologically and physically comfortable conditions must be provided for the individuals under study, and any random influences (psychological, physical, etc.) must be excluded.

14. Each time the measurements must be taken with filter and without it.

15. When the state of the individual is monitored by periodically taking the EPI-grams, the measurements must be taken at the same time of day, by the same physician, in the same room with constant optimum temperature, humidity and gas composition of the air, maintained by means of the ventilation and heating systems.

16. Factors which may interfere with the analysis:
* other diagnostic procedures being run concomitantly;
* medicines, natural substances and supplements;
* food intake (preferred to wait at least 3 hours after meals);
* smoking;
* alcohol and other drugs;
* menstruation in women.

17. For serial measurements, recurring registration of GDV-grams should be performed at the same time, by the same doctor, in the same room with constancy of temperature, humidity, air composition and maintenance thereof through ongoing ventilation and heating system controls.

18. It is necessary to establish comparable conditions of psychological and physical comfort for the patient, with specific attention to distractions and stressors; i.e. a   quiet, calming environment.

Part II. ELECTROPHOTONIC ANALYSIS IN THE INTEGRATIVE MEDICINE

Bioelectrographic Method for Preventive Health Care

From the early stage of bioelectrography development it was demonstrated that this approach may be applied in medicine in two main directions:

- Initial screening of patients which allows to detect main organs and systems of attention and direct patient to the next, more detailed and specific diagnostic techniques.
- Monitoring of patient's condition in the course of treatment and rehabilitation.

Both lines have been pursued by different research groups and we present some data published after the year 2000.

Photonic emission varies from person to person and reflects his/her psycho-emotional and physical state at the moment of study. Thus, bioelectrographic approach can then be used as a model to bridge the gaps in health disparities by creating an innovative approach to address health aspects in real time measurements, which will improve rural health outcomes. So very important question is: whether it is possible to use GDV approach for assessment of person's health state and psycho – physiological condition? This topic was the objective of the research by [Cohly H. et.al. 2009], and the aim was to create the dataset, which could serve as a background for an alternative method of preventive diagnostics based on impulse analysis of fingertips' photonic emission.

Pilot study encompasses 130 participants of average age of 25. The Integral area (IA), Integral entropy (IE) and activation coefficient (AC) mean values for 130 participants were recorded with and without filter. The relationship between IA, AC and IE was assessed by binary selection metric criteria. Specifically the average AC was 1.966 compared to the

29

standard norm ranging from 2 to 4, IA was ranging from 0.3 to 0.11 compared to the standard norm ranging from -0.6 to 1.0 whereas IE was ranging from 1.94 to 1.99 compared to the standard norm ranging from 1.0 to 2.0. Thus, pilot study of a group of 130 individuals shows close agreement with the values defined as a standard norm. Binary matrix analysis of the distribution of mean values is a promising step towards defining base line values for disease profiles. The participants with health problems showed deviation from the norm towards increased activity of certain organs.

This was confirmed in several studies.

Bundzen et al [2003] after analyzing 30 people concluded that basic and integral parameters of optoelectronic emission correlates with humoral-metabolic and reflex regulation processes on the level of the autonomic nervous system. Increase in activity of central (neurohumoral) part of auto-regulative mechanisms corresponds with the increase in the optoelectronic emission processes, increase of stress tolerance parameters, and an overall functional index, and corresponds with decrease in an index of energetic deficiency.

Several significant positive correlations for the DHEA and DHEA/cortisol values with several GDV measures of general health (area integer) and fourth finger for a group of people was found in [Dunlop 2004]. GDV left hand area values (both with and without filter) were significantly correlated to DHEA and DHEA/cortisol values. The GDV filter 4L finger entropy value, reflecting the energy condition of the endocrine system, was positively correlated with the cortisol value. The following GDV scores were positively correlated with the DHEA and DHEA/cortisol ratio: the right hand area integer (filter and non-filter), the filter right fourth finger entropy value, and both the left and right fourth finger area (no filter) change scores.

A proposed complex of diagnosis criteria using multiple diagnostic approaches can evaluate the organisms' response to therapy and assess the appropiateness of using different therapeutic influences. Using the GDV method in addition to other diagnostic approaches substantially simplifies (and speeds up) goal achievement – creating an individualized rehabilitation program and preventive recommendations [Voeikov 2004]

Classification of new patients by using a statistical model of GDV parameters coincided with the conventional classifications with an accuracy of 80%. Most information about the diseases in this experiment was derived from the finger sector -45° to 45° [Volkov 2005]..

The deviations of GDV-grams of the fingers revealed during some pathologic processes (107 people ages 18-62; 65 men, 42 women) do not always correspond to the borders of the sectors tentatively projected to particular organs or systems and quite often extend beyond these sector boundaries. For deviations showing post operative period increases, the majority of patients demonstrated disappearance of pathologic marks and restoration of integrity and saturation of energy field patterns [Kolkin 2006].

Kupeev et al [2006] after studding 73 people (ages 37-83; 31 men, 42 women) have concluded that GDV method can be used as an express-method for assessing treatment procedure effectiveness and persistency of acquired positive changes in organisms. GDV technique is quite sensitive and can detect changes in a few minutes.

Strong correlation between the GDV parameters and the diagnostic parameter measuring functional reserve capacity of a patient. This correlation has been revealed at its largest value for the filtered measures of GDV parameters on the left hand. The parameter "Number of fragments" shows large differences between ill and healthy patients at 6 of 10 fingers in the skin disease group [Gurski 2006] (328 patients).

Changes in organs and systems registered by the GDV method coincide in 60-90% of cases with changes registered by conventional diagnosis methods. Pathology initially detected by the means of GDV technique was confirmed afterwards by conventional methods in 60-70% of cases [Mamedov 2005] (more than 700 patients).

At the clinic of the Scientific Research Institute of Clinical and Experimental Lymphology of the Siberian Branch of the Russian Academy of Medical Sciences a double-blind screening examination of 100 verified patients with various pathologies demonstrated the sensibility of the GDV bioelectrography method amounted to 92% [Ignatiev et al 2000]. Examination of patients with autointoxication of various etiologies (diseases of the lymphatic system, of the digestive tract organs, etc) showed possibility to reveal and estimate the state of autointoxication by existence of markers - toxic spots of various kinds on bioelectrograms. Analysis of the data obtained from examination of 130 patients in hospital environment has proved that the bioelectrography method allows to reveal and estimate early before-clinical changes as well as hidden pathologic processes, which manifest themselves clinically later (with the period of observation from 1 month to 2 years) and are confirmed by laboratory and functional methods of research (cardiovascular pathology, diseases of endocrine, digestive, uro-genital systems and others).

Big research line was conducted at the Central Clinical Sanatorium named after F. Dzerzhinsky in Sochi, Russia, by Bikov A.T. M.D., PhD and Tchernousova L.D. M.D. [2003]. 135 people were examined with posttraumatic stress-factor disorders and 29 people with other anxiety-making disorders. 100% (164 people) of patients from these groups revealed somatic disfunction of their nervous system; 16.6% (27 people) of patients revealed changes in function of their endocrinic system-thyroid gland diseases; 11.1% (44 people) of patients revealed stomach and duodenum diseases (gastritis, duodenitis); 16.6% (27 people) of patients revealed diseases of biliferous tracts and pancreas (chronic cholecystitis, dyskinesia of biliferous tracts, reactive pancreatitis). GDV analysis of patients allowed to reveal dysfunctions not known by the previous investigations. Data presented in the Table below.

Table. Diseases revealed for the first time with the GDV method

Code	Name of disease	N of patients	%% out of number of patients
E00-E07	Diseases of thyroid gland i.a. goiter, euthereosis, autoimmune thyroiditis	29	5.6%
N40	Adenoma of prostate	7	1.3%
K80-K87	Diseases of bile cyst, biliferous tracts and pancreas	19	3.6%
K59	Functional disturbances of intestine (dysbacteriosis), chronic colitis	41	7.9%

All diagnoses were confirmed by clinical and laboratory examinations.

In the research project of phtisio-pulmonology department of Kazakh State Medical University named by S.D.Asfendiarov (Alma-Ata, Kazakhstan) 107 patients (60 men and 47 women) with lungs tuberculosis was studied both with GDV method and with classical technologies. 30

healthy people served as control [Shabaev et al 2004]. Clear statistical difference between healthy and deceased people, as well as high correlations (on the level 0.7-0.9) between GDV indexes and clinical parameters of patients were found. Another studied group included 195 patients (60% - women), bearer's of a profound mycosis fungoides infection - P. Variotii Bainier (1907), var. Zaaminella Dechkan (1974). Profound GDV-gram changes were noted in cases with eosinophilic reaction in blood correlated with anemia and decrease of immune status. These particularities could be connected with different biochemical basis of inflammation, but namely, with different stage of free-radical processes activation.

Monitoring of patents' condition after rehabilitation process is being used for many years since 2002 at the Centre of psychological research of Russian Ministry of Railway Transportation in Saint Petersburg [Sergeev et al 2004]. The short-term rehabilitation is designed for 6 hours. The doctor nominates necessary procedures depending on a condition of health and presence of problem zones, and traces changes after rehabilitation. After the ending procedures the card displaying dynamics of a condition (results of psychological diagnostics and the GDV analysis) is given out. After that results are discussing with the psychologist. After rehabilitation the GDV-gramms of fingers are characterized by the greater area, greater isolation and uniformity of a luminescence in relation to GDV-gramms before rehabilitation.

In this study correlation between GDV area and arterial pressure was found. Increase of arterial pressure corresponded to a smaller area of a luminescence (k = -0,320, p=0,01). Similar a pulse rate was correlated to the integrated area of a luminescence (k = -0.240, p=0.01), and pulse pressure (k = -0.272, p=0.01). The parameter of fractality without the filter had direct correlations with systolic (k= 0.325, p=0.01) and diastolic arterial pressure (k = 0.265, p=0.01). Increased fractality corresponded to increase of arterial pressure.

Interesting study was presented by [Abadi et al 2005]. They decided to compare informativeness of devices designed for measuring Human Energy Field. The four devices comprise: Gas Discharge Visualisation (GDV), Electro Scanning Method (ESM), Polycontrast Interference Photography (PIP) and Resonant Field Imaging (RFI). Each device delivers the information in different formats. Both RFI and ESM provide raw data (frequencies), which in the case of RFI is then used to build up an image, whereas in ESM no computer software is involved and the raw data is used in analysis. With PIP, the process of data collection and image creation is automated. GDV builds up an image based on readings taken at the fingertips.

10 participants were chance selected; each requested to complete a body perception questionnaire, in which they identified current and past health issues. The four scanning sessions for each participant took place on the same day and in the same order. The scans were interpreted by experts using qualitative analysis and compared to the health data from the client questionnaire.

Each of the devices has evidence from case studies, that has been able to demonstrate the possibility of identifying areas of physical and mental imbalance from scans. To date however only GDV has published research in peer review journals.

A blinded clinical study was performed by Prof. A.L. Tumanova at the Sochi University, Russia [Tumanova 2007], where 542 patients were separated in two groups. The first group was first analyzed with EPI /GDV and after that with ordinary medical examinations. The second group was first examined by a medical doctor and thereafter a EPI /GDV Analysis was done. The medical parameters included analysis of the cardio-vascular system with daily monitoring, of the bronchial system, the digestive tract, the spine and muscular system as well as blood, urine and hair tests. The study revealed a correlation of EPI /GDV Analysis Data with clinical examination for the first group between 82 and 89% and a predictive power of the EPI /GDV analysis prior to the medical examination of 94%. The correlation of the EPI /GDV Analysis with the results from the medical examinations for the second group (first medical examination and EPI /GDV Analysis afterwards) was 79%. The conclusion from this study was that the Analysis of EPI /EPI /GDV data was most gainful in cases of early diagnosis of pathological conditions. The advantages of the EPI /EPI /GDV approach were found in the ease in use, economical, fast, non-invasive, reliable and informative method of information gathering and diagnosis.

The meta-analysis of papers published in English or Russian language from 2003 to 2007 was presented in "The Journal of Alternative and Complementary Medicine". [Korotkov, Matravers et al 2010] "All randomized controlled studies (RCTs) and systematic research reports

(SRRs) were evaluated using Scottish Intercollegiate Guidelines Network and Jadad checklists. The search yielded 136 articles addressing four different fields of medical and psychophysiologic applications of EPI (GDV). Among them 78 were rated "high" on the two conventional checklists. **5303 patients** with different problems were compared to more than 1000 healthy individuals.

In the work by [Yakovleva et al 2008] correlations between parameters of the Ultrasonic Dopplerography of main brain arteries (USD MBA), Echocardiography (EchoCG) and Gas Discharge Visualization (GDV) were studied. 303 patients were examined by GDV and EchoCG methods and 43 patients by GDV and USD MBA.

Patients studied by USD of magisterial arteries of the head were divided to three groups in accordance with the level of vessels damage. Correlation analysis was done both for the whole set of subjects and for every particular group. For the whole group correlation between GDV and USD data was weak. For the particular groups correlations coefficients were moderate and strong with the level of significance $p < 0.05 - 0.01$. Different correlations were found both for all 10 fingers and for the sectors related to head zone at 1, 3 and 4 fingers; and in the sector of blood circulation. The highest correlations were noted at the first stages of the illness, that confirm the thesis of prognostic effectiveness of the GDV approach. Variations of vessels structure (stenoses, coilness, variation of diameter, etc.) were reflected on all GDV parameters. Presented results suggest existence of a linear dependence between data of Ultra-Sound Dopplerography of the magisterial arteries of the head and GDV parameters.

No linear correlations between Echocardiography and Gas Discharge Visualization (GDV) data were found.

The aim of the study [Ciesielska-Wrobel et al 2010] was to assess changes in EPI images in patients with cardiovascular diseases. The study population of 126 persons (81 men and 45 women) was divided into two groups: the study group consisted of 96 patients with coronary heart disease and the control group composed of 30 healthy persons. The study methods included recording of corona discharges of fingertips of both hands by using the Gas Discharge Visualization (GDV) Camera and analyzing changes in images dependent on conditions of medical examinations of patients, their frame of mind, age, gender, heart rate, blood pressure, serum potassium concentration, and the course of coronary heart disease.

Results: Age, gender, temperature in examination rooms as well as frame of mind of the study population exerted a similar effect on EPI in both groups. Heart rate, blood pressure and the pattern of coronary heart disease exerted varied effects on the patients' EPI parameters in the study group. Conclusions: The analysis of changes in EPI may be a source of information about the effect of physiological and pathophysiological changes in the human health state, physical as well as mental.

Detailed discussion of the principles of Electrophotonic analysis is presented in the book **"ENERGY FIELDS ELECTROPHOTONIC ANALYSIS IN HUMANS AND NATURE"** by K. Korotkov available in electronic format.

Bronchial Asthma

An analysis of the data which examines 247 patients with bronchial asthma (BA) compared to 56 practically healthy people was presented to demonstrate a practical medical application of gas discharge bioelectrography [Alexandrova R. et al, 2003, 2004]. In analyzing this group, a common trait distinguishing them was the pronounced liability of psychological status and vegetative instability. Significant correlations ($r > 0.5$, $p < 0.05$) were revealed between the indices of vegetative balance and parameters of the GDV-grams [Savitskaja G. 2001]. This was interpreted to confirm the contribution of the vegetative (autonomic) nervous system to the mechanisms of system energy-informational regulation. Good repeatability and reproducibility of the GDV-grams' parameters were found for the absolute majority of the investigated healthy people and BA patients (in 90% of the cases).

The GDV-grams of a practically healthy individual with basal metabolism and in harmony with the environment (i.e. non-stressful situation), is characterized by a uniform fluorescent corona located as the middle ring of the GDV diagram.

The GDV-gram of a patient with BA attack is distinguished by an 'outburst' of glow in the respiratory zone of the fifth finger. At the same time this notion has a non-specific character as a similar 'outburst' of glow in the respiratory zone of the fifth finger may be detected in a patient with a left-side pneumonia.

Average values of indices of the GDV-gram in the groups of patients and healthy people are given in table 1.

Table 1. Average values of the GDV-gram parameters in the groups of patients and healthy people. Parameters of GDV images: FC – form coefficient; FrC – fractal coefficient; EC – emission coefficient.

Groups of the investigated people	GDV parameters			
	FC	FrC	EC	Area
1. BA patients	132.8 +/− 29.5	10.8 +/− 2.41	1.23 +/− 0.11	6740 +/− 651.7
2. Patients with stomach and duodenum ulcer	109.9 +/− 24.4	8.9 +/− 1.84	2.5 +/− 0.26	8450 +/− 817.0
3. Healthy people	93.8 +/− 20.9	7.47 +/−.67	0.48 +/-05	10869 +/− 1051.1
Statistics	Н́	Н́	$P_{1-2} < 0.001$ $P_{2-3} < 0.001$	$P_{1-3} < 0.05$

Diagnostically most informative are the indices which characterize the area of GDV-gram. As we see from table 1, area values for healthy people are always greater, as compared to that of unhealthy patients. For the BA group the GDV area is larger in proportion to greater severity cases, higher degrees of pulmonary obstruction and more pronounced dysfunctions of the microcirculation in the lungs as seen in diagnostic scintigraphic data. Emission coefficients (EC) statistically differ between the groups, as well, while fractal coefficients (FC and FrC) demonstrate less significant difference.

The GDV-gram of BA patients both overall, and in the rehabilitation period after acute exacerbation is characterized by lower values of area indices and the area integral coefficient (JgS) as compared to practically healthy people. JgS values for healthy people are $0.56^{238}_{99}.35$ on the left and $0.54^{238}_{99}.33$ on the right, whereas for BA patients $0.42^{238}_{99}.64$ on the left hand and $0.51^{238}_{99}.69$ on the right hand (P=0.01). The conjugacy of JgS changes can be revealed in sector or zone analysis by correlations with the respiratory meridian notion in Traditional Chinese Medicine. Table 2 demonstrates the difference in JgS average value in these zones, which do, and do not correspond to the respiratory system. Table 3 illustrates a significant correlations between JgS values in the zones for respiratory systems.

38

Table.2 Difference of JgS average values of zones, which correspond* and which do not correspond to the respiratory system for BA patients (n=122)

	Zones	JgS value	Statistics
1	Transverse colon'	**0.07**	$P_{1-2} < 0.01$
2	Small intestine	0.39	
3	Thorax zone of spine'	**0.07**	$P_{3-4} < 0.001$
4	Sacrum	0.5	
5	Respiratory system	**0.07**	$P_{5-6} < 0.001$
6	Kidneys	0.52	

Table.3 Coefficients of correlation of JgS values in the zones, corresponding to the respiratory system for BA patients (n=122)

Zones	Transverse colon	Thorax zone of spine	Respiratory system
Transverse colon		0.69 $p < 0.0001$	0.65 $p < 0.0001$
Respiratory system	0.65 $p < 0.0001$	0.61 $p < 0.0001$	

This data confirms the clinical significance and high correlation for sector diagnostics in the analysis of the GDV-grams.

Monitoring of the dynamics of change of GDV-gram's parameters applying one-time medical treatment and in the process of course therapy.

Observations pre and post daily therapy as well as day-to-day monitoring via GDV-grams could detect substantive changes which correlate with the clinical course and effects of both medications and treatment modalities. In several instances it was able to forecast possible side effects of therapy. Correlations were able to be established between GDV-patterns' transformations and the dynamics of leading pathogenetic processes for BA patients, including external respiratory dysfunction, microcirculation in the lungs, and other markers of bronchial inflammatory processes [Alexandrova et. al., 2001].

GDV parameters register demonstrated reliable differences on the influence of glucocorticosteroids relative to the ways of their injection: positive under inhalation and inhibitory under intravenous infusion. This significant depression of bioenegetic activity due to intravenous infusions suggests yet another rationale for limiting its application as a type of therapy so as to avoid side effects systemically from treatment.

Noteworthy was the positive influence in bioenergetic activity measures for the patient after a course of medical acupuncture. Reliable increase of JgS in the process of reflexotherapy preceded positive functional shifts in clinical treatment outcome. Speculation that energy-informational regulation of the patient 's activity is one of the main mechanisms for the acupuncture effect observed.

Yet another modality, the homeopathic medication "Pumpan" administered to 22 BA patients with cor pulmonale rendered positive and clinically distinct energy-informational effects relative to both 'placebo' and inhibitory agents such as Nitrosorbid. Improvements in bioenergetic activity for patients was noted within two hours after Pumpan, and accompanied by the increase of peak speed of expiration (p<0.01), decrease in right atrium burden, and improvement of the process of repolarization of the heart ventricles with diffusive character (p<0.05). These studies using GDV bioelectrography gave further evidence for the recommendation that Pumpan be used as an additional remedy for complex treatment approaches for BA patients with the subset of cor pulmonale.

In another clinical application, GDV techniques performed on 70 BA patients with pathologic gastroduodenum zone findings (e.g. erosive gastroduodenitis, stomach and duodenum ulcer) reflected changes on the system character of inflammation of mucous membranes of patients - atopics with a characteristic energy-informational exchange. This analysis demonstrated similarity in the dynamics of an inflammatory process shared by both the bronchi and the gastroduodenum zones. Moreover, a result of the GDV technique for this group of patients provided further energetic support for the use of acupuncture as a method to reverse and rebalance both conditions. Complex therapy with the application of acupuncture for BA patients with pathology of gastroduodenum zone was accompanied by a more pronounced improvement of patency of airways, the decrease of levels of the bronchi inflammation markers, and recovery of the disturbed balance of energy exchange according to BE data ($p < 0.05$).

Conclusion. Patterns of GDV-grams of fingers from BA patients correlate with known main pathogenic identifiers giving evidence of the clinical usefulness, informativeness of BE and its complementary role in clinical medicine. Introduction of this GDV technique into the medicine practice for BA considerably widens the objective diagnostics and clinical monitoring capabilities of the patient's global state; moreover, its use contributes to greater individualization of therapeutic options. An obvious result of this work is in its application to the study of mechanisms and outcomes for both traditional medical remedies as well as an array of complementary strategies such as acupuncture and homeopathy.

Similar conclusions was made in the research of big group of BA patients by Vilner N.S. and Spizina E.A. [2002].

Autistic children analysis

Similar approach was used for detecting heterogeneity and unique features in autism [Kostyuk N. et.al. 2009, 2010].

The autistic children in this study were previously diagnosed with mild autism and/or Asperger's Syndrome. The age of the autistic children fell into a range of five to twelve years old, 9.3 being the mean age. All autistic participants were males. To reduce the barrier of a new setting for autistic children, parents were asked to participate first. The cerebral cortex, cerebral vessels, spleen, epiphysis, left kidney, gallbladder, abdomen, sacrum and thorax show lower activity compared to the rest of the organs.

Results revealed heterogeneity and unique features in the participants with ASD and their parents. The low activities that were found in the zones of gastro-intestinal tract, immune system, cerebral cortex, and cerebral vessels have been described in the literature and confirm previous data on autistic patients. These zones were found to be present in all autistic children we tested and therefore are unique signatures of autism in our preliminary study. Additionally, the bio-electrographic study detected epiphysis, kidneys, adrenal gland, cervical zone, thorax zone and sacrum as the zones of misbalance in autistic children. Despite of being diagnosed with Asperger's syndrome/mild autism, autistic children had different values assigned to the zones of cerebral cortex and cerebral vessels. This indicates that there exists heterogeneity within one phenotype which implies the individualized approach. The uneven distribution of EPE especially as to the response of the parasympathetic nervous system leads us to hypothesize that there exists a misbalance, which is expressed on the physical level in respective zones of EPE.

Brothers and sisters of the autistic children though labeled as normals also exhibited unique features common to autistic sibling but additionally had low activities in pancreas and pelvis minor zone. The only difference between the autistic children and their siblings is in the distribution of EPE values. In autistic children the distribution is very uneven between left and right hand while in the siblings the distribution is fairly even.

The fathers of the autistic children share some unique features of autism such as cerebral cortex, cerebral vessels, epiphysis and spleen. Characteristically fathers show low activities in the liver, transverse colon, descending colon, respiratory system, cardiovascular system and coronary vessels.

Mothers of the autistic children share some unique features of autism such as cerebral cortex, cerebral vessels, immune system, epiphysis and kidneys. Distinguishing features include transverse colon, pancreas, and urogenital system. The images were characterized by inconsistency and gaps pertaining to certain sector. The outer isoline of some images had fractile nature which could be the evidence of emotional tension or stress.

In conclusion, bioelectrographic method is a promising step towards creating autism profile and identifying unique signatures pertaining to the parents and their siblings. Further work should involve more participants in order to augment our findings by the bioelectrographic approach.

A correlation between GDV and heart rate variability measures

This study [Cioca G, et.al. 2004] was an extension of the studies previously presented [Bundzen, 2002; Korotkov, 2002; Buyantseva, 2003]. The control subjects (n=24) from that study were volunteers from the State Medical Academy in Russia and were used for the Orthostatic test. Fourty-three athletes (age 19-24) from the State Research Institute of Sport in Russia volunteered for the exercise tests.

Heart Rate Variability (HRV). HRV measures were recorded using a traditional electrocardiogram with four leads attached to the left + right hands and the left + right ankles. HRV was calculated using the NeuroSoft Company (Russia) and Polar Electro (Finland) Software. Heart Rate (HR) was calculated using following formula: $HR = 60 \times 10^3$ msec/R-R, where R-R is the average length in seconds of the R-R intervals (RRNN) for each group. Two parameters were calculated from the time domain measures of R-R interval variability. The standard deviation of R-R intervals (SDNN) can be used as a measure of sympathetic nervous activity, whereas the root-mean square of successive differences in R-R intervals (RMSSD) reflects parasympathetic activity.

Spectral analysis of time domain curves reveals peaks in the very low frequency range (VLF: 0.004-0.04 Hz), the low-frequency range (LF: 0.04-0.15 Hz) and the high frequency range (HF: 0.15-0.5 Hz). LF/HF is the ratio of the low / high frequency power components. The VLF parameter is believed to measure the hormonal regulation (with some sympathetic nervous system activity), the LF parameter is a measure of the sympathetic nervous system and the HF parameter is a measure of the activity of the parasympathetic system.

Background HRV and GDV measures were taken after 5 minutes of resting in a quiet room. In addition HRV and GDV measures were also taken following the three experimental conditions. For the Orthostatic test, subjects were asked to deep breathe in a supine position for 5 minutes (controlled breathing involved 6 breaths per minute with 5 second inhalations and 5 second exhalations). Then subjects stood up and resumed regular tidal breathing. After 5 minutes GDV and HRV measures were obtained.

The exercise test involved 10 minutes of strenuous physical exercise before GDV and HRV measures were obtained. The third experimental condition was the consumption of dark chocolate, three hours after which GDV and HRV measures were taken. Correlation coefficients were calculated for GDV and HRV results obtained during the background and during the three experimental conditions. In addition to analysis of individual sessions, the difference between the orthostatic and background tests was calculated. Significant correlations were seen using GDV parameters from individual fingers (eg 5R), for differences between two fingers (eg. 5L-5R) or by using all 10 fingers (eg. deviations in absolute values, or mathematical combinations of all ten (stress index). Two GDV parameters (stress index and area) correlate with a balanced sympathetic and parasympathetic regulation of HRV. The same balanced regulatory state has been previously reported for other positive emotional stimuli (McCraty, 1995).

In the present study, despite the parasympathetic dominance associated with exercise, the sympathetic component of HRV (LF) was correlated with the stress index parameter of GDV. Thus the sympathetic nervous activity appears to best correlate with GDV parameters in two different experimental conditions controlled by either sympathetic or parasympathetic activity.

In conclusion HRV and GDV were correlated in a non-diseased population under different physiological conditions. In situations where either the sympathetic or the parasympathetic nervous systems were activated, the HRV parameter corresponding to sympathetic regulation of heart rate was correlated with GDV. In a situation inducing a positive emotional state, the HRV parameter which correlates with GDV is the balance between the sympathetic and parasympathetic nervous systems. In all cases, GDV entropy correlated with the different HRV parameters. Since these HRV parameters reflect involuntary reactions of the heart to psycho-physical loading, the observed correlation between HRV and GDV allows the conclusion that well being can be measured as a resilience to psycho-physical stimuli.

In another research 60 athletes in the age of from 18 till 23 years, among them 30 wrestlers of high qualification took part [Lovygina 2005]. GDV and HRV parameters were measured both in initially and after the loading. Significant correlations between respiratory waves (RW) and GDV area (r = - 0.70 p < 0.05) and sluggish waves of the 1st order (SW-1) (r = - 0.69 p < 0.05) was found.

Surgery

For several years research project for evaluation of patients' condition after surgery was conducted in Saint Petersburg Military Medical Academy. A lot of papers were published in Russian medical journals and two PhD in medicine were awarded. Two papers were published in English [Polushin et.al. 2004, 2009]. The main conclusions were as follows:

1.   There are reliable differences between parameters of GDV-grams of practically healthy people and patients with chronic abdominal surgical pathology.

2.   The data obtained indicate that GDI parameters are connected with the functional status of the organism and reflect the severity of the somatic state of patients with abdominal surgical pathology.

3.   The most informative parameters are: "integral area of glow JS" in the "GDV Diagram" program; "total" and "normalized area", "total density", "average brightness", as well as "fractality" and "form coefficient" in the "GDV Processor" program.

4.   The most informative mode of registration of GDV-grams is the mode "without filter". On the whole, the application of the filter keeps the trend of changes, but they are often less pronounced and lose statistical significance.

5.   The revealed variability of GDV-gram parameters depending on the sex and age of patients indicates that it is necessary to determine their individual norms.

6.   The dependence of perioperative dynamics of a number of indices on the severity of the patient's somatic state, the patient's age and the duration of surgical procedure enables functional monitoring in the postoperative period, and evaluation of operative stress.

7.   The parameters of EPI-grams reliably change in response to the operative trauma, and their dynamics depend on the severity of the somatic state of patient, which allows using the technique for functional monitoring of patients in postoperative period, as well as for the assessment of the operative stress. The degree of intensity of changes depended on the volume and character of the undergone physical intervention. Thus, patients who had laparoscopic cholecystectomy showed much smaller changes of bioenergy status in comparison with patients, who had stomach and intestine's operations.

8.   The Electrophotonic Imaging technique is mostly advisable for the dynamic assessment of the functional state of patient in perioperative period. Not all the fingers may be used, at that, but only one finger of each hand. For example, the fourth finger, where the changes are the most significant.

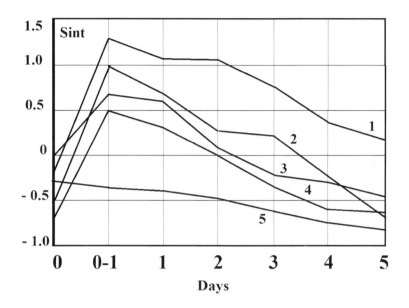

Dynamics of GDV-gram parameters of systems in perioperative period.
0 – before surgery, 0-1 – first hour after surgery, 1-5 days after surgery.
Curves 1-4 – favorable prognosis; 5 – unfavorable prognosis.

Important approach for monitoring of GDV parameters to predict the development of postoperative delirium was developed by Strukov EU. and Tuzhikova N.V. [2010].

122 people were surveyed using a prospective GDV technique. Three groups were examined. The first (control) were 47 healthy people surveyed by GDV against the background of psycho-emotional well-being. The second group included 50 patients operated on the abdominal organs. GDV-grams were recorded in the group before surgery and during the next five days postoperatively. The third group consisted of 25 patients treated at the clinic of psychiatry with the abstinent syndrome in pre-and delirious state. The most informative was glow area parameter. In series taken in dynamics the most significant changes were revealed. Dynamics

of the glow area parameter of patients, whose postoperative period is complicated by the development of delirium, is different from the normal distribution and was characterized by high amplitude of the GDV area. Dynamic changes in the glow area were similar to the dynamics of GDV images of patients with psychiatric profile. However, these changes in the operated patients may be revealed 10-12 hours prior to the development of the clinical picture of delirium. As the delirious syndrome subsided, the parameter of GDV area comes-back to the original data and fits into the standard distribution. Such performance of dynamics of the GDV area and its fundamental similarity to that of patients with psychiatric profile allows us to speak with confidence about the possibility of prognosis of delirious syndrome in patients operated on the abdominal organs in the immediate postoperative period, even before the development of complications.

Evaluation of disturbed uteroplacental blood circulation in the course of Pregnancy

Big research project was conducted in Rostov Federal Research Institute of Obstetrics and Pediatrics [Gimbut 2000, 2004]. The aim of the study was to evaluate informative diagnostic criteria of normal and pathological flow of pregnancy. Practically all the types of pregnancy distress are characterized by the disturbed blood circulation of the "mother – placenta – fetus" system. 226 pregnant women were examined in I and II trimesters of pregnancy. The author used special method of evaluation:

The average thickness of corona in the uterus sector of the ring finger of each hand was measured under negative and positive polarity of the electrical field. The coefficient of disbalance (CD) was calculated for each hand according to the following formula:

$$CD = 3\tfrac{3}{2}(Tp - Tn) / D,$$

where Tp – average thickness of corona in the uterus sector under positive polarity of the electromagnetic field, mm; Tn – average thickness of corona in the uterus sector under negative polarity of electromagnetic field, mm; D – longitudinal diameter of the finger circle in the photograph, mm.

The following conclusions were presented by the author:

1. The developed modification of GDV technique demonstrated an informative and stable GDV parameter – the coefficient of disbalance.

2. The coefficient of disbalance for acupuncture points associated with the uterus is a highly specific and highly sensitive indicator for the course of pregnancy:

a) regardless of the period of gestation, stably low CD GDV parameters correspond to the normal course of pregnancy – the coefficient of disbalance tends to zero for both hands.

b) when the parameters of utero- and feto-placental blood flow deviate from the normative values, the CD reliably increases for one hand.

c) under the danger of miscarriage, regardless of the period of gestation, the CD is higher for both hands as compared to the norm.

d) the stimulation of EP-147 point under the danger of miscarriage, simultaneously with the normalization of parameters of uterine blood flow, leads to reliable decrease of the CD down to the normal values.

di)

3.   There exists an inversely proportional correlation between the CD of acupuncture points associated with the uterus and the intensity of gestational dominant. Low values of the CD correspond to the manifested characteristics of the gestational dominant; the CD parameters are reliably higher when the gestational dominant weakens.

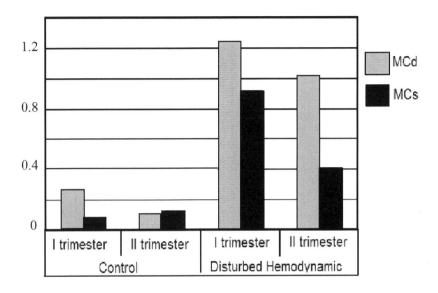

Fig. GDV parameters in case of normal pregnancy and pregnancy complication. MCd and MCs - misbalance coefficient in the uterine sector on the right (dexter) and left (sinister) hands, accordingly.

Hyrudo-Therapy Treatment

Leech therapy is an ancient method of natural treatment developed in India several thousand years ago and very popular in Russia. Professor Albert Krashenuk is a great proponent of leech treatment and he conducted several research projects to verify the method [Krashenuk et al 2004, 2006]. He is using GDV instrument in his everyday practice.

For the statistical analysis 240 patients were selected, including 56 men (23,3%) and 184 women (76,7%). They were measured with GDV instrument before and several times in the process of hyrudotherapy treatment. All patients demonstrated statistically significant positive transformation of their Energy Field: increase of Area, decrease of Fractality, which created uniform, solid Energy Field. This process had several stages, quite typical for a whole series of patients, which allowed proposing a hypothesis on trigger character of observed effects of leeches, which cause specific reactions in the organism of patients. Thus, that involves the change of GDV glow and classical parameters, registered by other techniques.

Fig demonstrates the statistically significant effects of hyrudotherapy treatment to people of different age. As we see from this diagram both increase and decrease of the HEF Area may be observed which in most cases may be interpreted as normalization of energy condition. For more than 85% of people this effect was statistically significant.

This effect was tested in the experiment with white laboratory rats. 10 selected rats of the same breed were randomly divided to two groups. During several sessions for every rat in one group a leach was applied for 10 minutes while for rats in another group 10 ml of blood were pumped out with syringe. GDV parameters from the rat tail were measured 1 and 2 hours after the procedure. As we see from the graphs in the first three procedures the difference between experimental and control groups was statistically significant (the level of variations is about 13-15%) while after a month there were no difference. This confirms data of multiple observations that leach therapy has significant influence for the people having problems and practically no influence to healthy organisms.

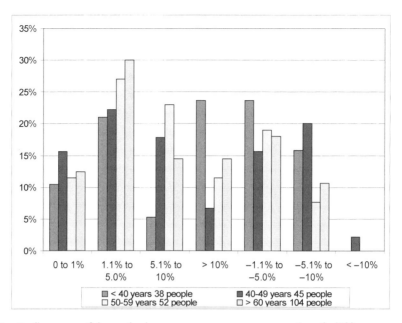

Fig. Influence of hyrudotherapy treatment to people of different age.

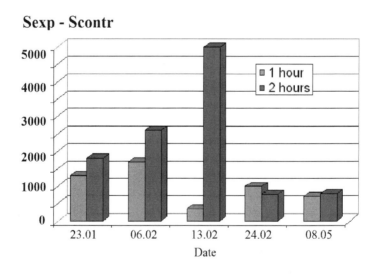

Fig. Relative changes of the GDV Area for the control and experimental groups of rats 1 and 2 hours after blood drawing-off for control group and leach sucking for experimental group.

Oncology

For many years in Georgian National Institute of Oncology GDV instrument was used for analysis of patients. Possibility of evaluation of cancer process at early stages and monitoring patients' condition in the process of treatment was demonstrated. Several papers were published [Vepkhvadze 2003; Gagua 2003, 2006; Gedevanishvili 2004] and it was very well accepted by medical professionals, but research was not supported by any grunts due to the bad economical situation in Georgia and Russian-Georgian political tension in mid-2000. Let us look to some results of this work.

For the statistical analysis the following subjects diagnosed with III stage of cancer 109 subjects of both genders with lung cancer and 140 women with breast cancer were selected; control group consisted of 44 practically healthy people and 54 women with different non-oncological conditions. All patients were diagnosed with cancer by conventional means including biopsy; GDV measures were taken from 10 fingers of both hands before any oncology treatment and 2 and 6 weeks after complex treatment including surgery, chemotherapy, irradiation and CAM psycho-rehabilitation. Blind study design.

Statistically significant difference between GDV parameters of oncology patients and non-oncology groups was found for all studied cases. After treatment statistical trend of GDV parameters towards healthy population parameters was revealed. Example of experimental data is presented at fig.. The conclusion was that GDV Technique presents objective measures for evaluation of cancer state and monitoring the patient's condition after treatment. The method is easy for application, non-invasive, objective and cheap. From several years of experience a good potential for the development of a method of early evaluation of the probability of potential cancer is clearly seen. This approach should be based on computer data-mining multiparametric comparison with database of nosological cases.

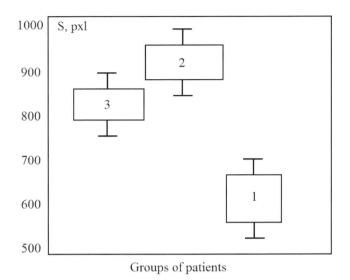

Fig. Averaged GDV Areas for the groups of patients with breast cancer before (2) and after (3) combined treatment and group of practically healthy women (1). Data are taken from the finger 5L.

Electrophotonic approach to early diagnosis of Polyps and Colon Cancer was offered by Saeidov [2010]. Analysis by GDV- measurements and monitoring of the states of people with polyps in the colon and cancer of the transverse colon revealed a definite pattern in correspondence of the GDV parameters to changes in parts of the colon and their development in time. The correlation between the glow shape of the GDV sector of colon and polyps on the corresponding portion of the colon has been revealed. The parameter, sensitively responsive to the emergence and growth of polyps in the colon has been determined. A long-term GDV monitoring of the patient with a cancerous tumor in the transverse colon showed more than 40% of the "normalized intensity" parameter of the part of colon with tumor after 4 years of observations. A parametric difference and temporal parameters dynamics of the whole body and parts of the colon during the emergence and growth of polyps and the presence of tumor have been established.

Results of using the GDV technique in monitoring process of complex treatment of patients with colon cancer was presented in

[Kartashova et al 2007]. Patients were 3 women and 7 men 55+/-10 years old suffering from colon cancer of stage 2-3 and having surgery and chemotherapy. For 82% of patients in post-operative period energy deficiency in immune and endocrine systems, cerebral zone and colons were recorded. In rehabilitation period 75% of patients demonstrated gradual increase of Energy Field with suppression of immune and endocrine systems. In 25% of patients energy parameters had tendency to deterioration, which correlated with clinical parameters: increase of cancer antigen and deterioration of biochemical parameters.

In the Russian Research Center of Radiology and Surgery Technologies research project was developed under the guidance of Professor Gennady Garinov [Garinov and Korotkov 2012]. 100 patients diagnosed with prostate cancer (PC) with conventional means including biopsy; and having conventional treatment have been selected for the study. All men, aged 63+/-15 years old. All participants voluntary agreed to take part in the research and were informed of the procedures and expected outcomes. Based on the results of the PSA analysis and clinical observations participants were distributed to three groups: "negative prognosis", "positive prognosis" and "intermediate prognosis". GDV measures were taken from 10 fingers of both hands before 2 - 6 weeks after complex treatment including surgery, chemotherapy and irradiation. Blind study design. Preliminary studies demonstrated that certain integral GDV characteristics of patients with prostate cancer correlated with the clinical course of malignant process. A comparison of the characteristics of GDV and the growth rate of prostate cancer also indicates the close relationship between these parameters. Statistically significant difference between GDV parameters of patients with positive and negative prognosis of PC was found.

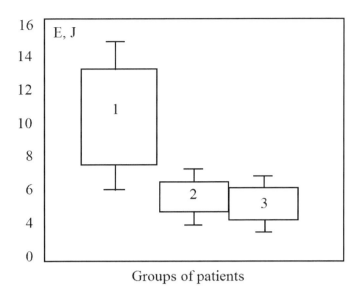

Fig. Statistical distribution of EPI parameters of PC patients divided to three groups in accordance with the rate of tumor development: fast growing (1), stagnant (3), and intermediate (2).

Discussion of the peculiarities of cancer analysis may be found in the book by Korotkov K.G. «Energy fields Electrophotonic analysis in humans and nature». 2012. e-book: Amazon.com.

Diabetes

Research of 2 type diabetic patients was done at the Arogyadhama, a holistic health home, Bangalore, India by Bhawna Sharma [2012]. Total of 79 male (mean age 59.71 ± 11.03) and 68 female (mean age 56.38 ± 9.15) participated in the study. Mean year of diabetes history were, 9.40 ± 7.41. This group was again divided into three groups according to year of diabetes history, **Dia1** (diabetes history <= 5 years), **Dia2** (5 years < diabetes history <= 10 years) and **Dia3** (>10 years diabetes history). 89 apparently healthy people (mean age 56.39 ± 9.27) served as control.

Left-right hand energy coefficient imbalance 4L-4R (fourth finger on left and right hand) have shown significant differences (p = 0.034). In GDV screening software diabetes group was significantly different from the normal group on cardiovascular, endocrine, digestive, urinogenital systems at p<0.01 and on nervous and immune systems at p<0.05. Normal groups showed significant difference when compared with Dia2 and Dia3 at endocrine, urinogenital and immune systems. No significant difference was noticed between Dia1 and normal groups. Dia1 was significantly different from Dia2 and Dia3 at immune system.

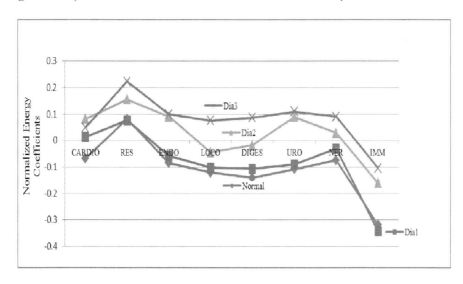

Fig. EPI parameters distribution for different groups.

After subtracting normal group mean from diabetes group mean, out of 30 organs or organ systems from GDV diagram 12 showed increasing trend from Dia1 to Dia3 groups (see Table below). Out of these 12 organs 5 organs acupuncture points are located on ring finger, i.e. 4L and 4R (underlined at the graph). Four variables, cardiovascular system, coronary vessels, epiphysis and hypophysis showed similar values (more than 0.1) of deviation of normalised energy coefficient of different diabetes groups from the normal group. Acupuncture points, epiphysis and hypophysis are also located on ring fingertip.

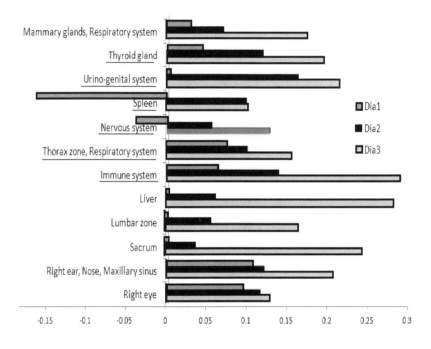

Fig. Data for 3 diabetes groups after subtracting Normal mean from different diabetes group means.

As we see from these data there is present clear statistical difference both between apparently healthy population and diabetes groups and between groups with different level of diabetes. This may allow to create diagnostic model for evaluation the probability of the diabetes development. This may be even done based on measurements only two ring fingers. We can imaging the value of this approach would it be able to substitute existing diabetes tester based on blood test.

Statistical model of patients' diagnosis based on GDV parameters

A statistical model based on GDV parameters of the patients which allowed diagnosing the patient disease with a certain probability was developed [Volkov et al 2005]. To construct the model, with- and without-filter GDV-grams from 177 patients with known diseases were studied. All patients were classified into 6 groups according to their actual diagnoses:

- Group "Normal" (persons with relatively good health)
- Group "Diseases of blood circulation"
- Group "Diseases of endocrine system"
- Group "Diseases of digestive apparatus"
- Group "Diseases of musculoskeletal system"
- Group "Other diseases," comprising diseases different from listed above.

As the result of processing GDV-grams in the program *GDV Scientific Laboratory*, the average (over all fingers) values of following GDV parameters were obtained:

- Image area
- Coefficient of the image form (measure of the GDV symmetry)
- Average radius of isoline
- Isoline radius deviation from its average value
- Isoline length
- Entropy along the isoline (measure of the image disorder)
- Average intensity
- Number of image fragments
- Fractality along the isoline (measure of the image complexity)
- Fractality deviation from its average value

The same parameters but within 4 sectors of finger image were also calculated, including sectors 1 (-45°, 45°), 2 (45°, 135°), 3 (135°, 225°), and 4 (225°, 315°). This was done to statistically test the hypothesis that various finger sectors could be related to different features of the organism.

The statistical discriminant analysis of the GDV parameters from combinations of the parameters from the first sector were found which allowed to classify the patients into groups almost coinciding with the actual groups related to their diagnoses. Namely, the classification of the patients by using the model based on the GDV parameters from the first sector had coincided with the actual classification with the accuracy of 75−85%. In other words, taking an arbitrary patient from the groups of known diseases and analyzing only his/her GDV parameters in the first sector, we can predict the group with the probability of 75−85%.

The constructed statistical model was verified on new 94 patients having the same diseases. No information from these patients was used during the model formation; therefore, the model run on the new patients was a necessary independent test. The classification of the new patients by using the model coincided with the actual classification with the accuracy of 80%. This result can be regarded as good, and it raises the statistical significance of the model.Using the results of the study, we may conclude that most information about the diseases listed in the beginning is stored in the finger sector (-45°, 45°).

Presented ideas were developed by this group and presented next year [Gursky 2006]. The following normalization procedure was used to set values of all GDV parameters at a uniform scale. Each GDV parameter value at each finger of a patient was divided by the parameter average over all fingers. In each disease group, mean deviations of the normalized GDV parameters from their group average values were analyzed. The idea was to compare these deviations (dispersion) with those in the group of conventionally healthy patients, who were the patients without the disease considered. For diagnostic aims, an informative case would be if the mean deviation of some GDV parameter in the group with a disease was smaller enough than that in the group without the disease. The following diseases were analyzed for the purpose:

$\frac{35}{17}$ Diseases of gastrointestinal tract as the main syndrome (94 patients)

$\frac{35}{17}$ Diseases of cardiovascular system (81 patients)

$\frac{35}{17}$ Skin diseases (41 patients)

The method of neural networks was used to create models in which various sets of the GDV parameters served as the input parameters. The model output was the categorical parameters defining a class of functional states which a patient belongs to. The model was derived on the overall sample of patients, which was divided into three samples: training sample (about 80% of all patients), cross-validation sample (about 20%), and test sample (about 20%).

The parameter "Reserve" quantifies states of increased and decreased internal functional reserve of organism. The results of the neural net model based on the filter GDV parameters at the left hand, obtained on the training and control samples are presented in the Table.

Model / Fact Training Samples	Group "Decreased Reserve"	Group "Increased Reserve"
Correct	**57**	**62**
Wrong	17	14
% of correctly classified patients	**77%**	**82%**
Model / Fact Test Samples	Group "Decreased Reserve"	Group "Increased Reserve"
Group "Decreased Reserve"	19	16
Group "Increased Reserve"	7	6
% of correctly classified patients	**73%**	**73%**

As we see from this Table, the percentage of right classification was more than 73%.

The analysis of the normalized GDV parameters dispersion in groups with diseases of gastrointestinal tract, cardiovascular system, and skin had shown that the maximal difference between parameters deviations in groups of conventionally ill and conventionally healthy is of 20–30%. The maximal difference was demonstrated by parameter "Number of fragments" (up to 39%;).

These results on GDV parameters average deviations can be helpful for the diagnostics process. New patient can be assigned to the risk group for a particular disease with a certain probability if his/her values of the GDV parameters lie in specific ranges.

Unfortunately, due to different reasons this model had no further development, but this work demonstrated possibility to develop system of automatic diagnosis based on GDV parameters. This line was successfully developed by a group led by Dr Ekaterina Jakovleva.

Electrophotonic Analysis of Arterial Hypertension

For several years research on bioelectrography application for patients with Arterial Hypertension (AH) was conducted in Russian National Research Medical University named after N.I. Pirogov, Moscow and in Federal Medical and Biological Agency, Moscow. Big group of medical doctors conducted the study: Elena V. Aleksandrova M.D., Tatiana V. Zarubina M.D., Margarita N. Kovelkova M.D., Ph.D., Peter V.Strychkov M.D., Ph.D., Ekaterina G. Yakovleva M.D., Ph.D. [Yakovleva EG et al 2006, 2008; Aleksandrova EV et al 2010, 2011; Korobko IE et al 2012]. Reliable differences between the control group (healthy patients) and groups with various degrees and stages of AH were calculated with sufficiently high accuracy which allowed to include Electrophotonic - Gas Discharge Visualization technique into the mass-population screening.

Several classifications of arterial hypertension are accepted in medicine. To date, according to UHO recommendations arterial hypertension is classified into 3 degrees (depending on the degree of AP elevation) and 3 stages (depending on the involvement of target organs). There are also 4 categories of arterial hypertension depending on the likelihood of cardio-vascular complications in the nearest 10 years. The complications are related to the presence of the risk-factors, involvement of target organs and/or concomitant (associated) diseases.

The study was aimed at:

1. Calculating discriminative functions to detect patients with different degrees and stages of arterial hypertension as well as the risk of cardio-vascular complications; assessing dependence of the most qualitative patient grouping on one of the recognized AH classifications.
2. Assessing the influence of patients' gender on calculation discriminative functions.
3. Building the model of logistic regression to detect patients with different degrees of AH severity.

Materials and methods

603 patients aged from 18 to 83, 265 males and 338 females served as participants. All were divided into groups according to AH degree and stage and degree of cardio-vascular complications risk in the nearest 10 years. Groups were divided as follows:

Control group – 136 people (47 men and 89 women) and experimental group – 467 people (218 men and 249 women).

Experimental group was in its turn divided in different ways:

According to the degree of AH: AH1 of the 1st degree – 92 persons (38 men and 54 women); AH2 of the 2nd degree – 185 people (89 men and 96 women); AH3 of the 3d degree – 190 people (91 men and 99 women).

According to the AH stage: AHs1 of the 1st stage – 103 people (40 men and 63 women); AHs2 of the 2nd stage – 283 people (130 men and 153 women); AHs3 of the 3d stage – 81 persons (48 men and 33 women).

According to the likely risk of cardio-vascular complications: low risk (risk 1) – 56 people (24 men and 32 women); moderate risk (risk 2) – 88 people (33 men and 55 women); high risk (risk 3) – 114 people (51 men and 63 women); extremely high risk (risk 4) – 209 people (110 men and 99 women).

In the course of the study the following EPI /GDV-gram parameters were analyzed: image area, normalized area, intensity, spectrum width, brightness and fractality. According to these parameters we analyzed images of all 10 fingers as a whole as well as of separate sectors selected in accordance with Korotkov's Diagnostic Table: cerebral cortex, cerebral vessels, the right and left heart, vascular system, coronary vessels, hypophysis, hypothalamus, epiphysis, thyroid, suprarenals, kidneys, the nervous system. Organs and systems of organs which were involved in the onset and progress of arterial hypertension were under consideration.

All data were processed with the "GDV-Processor" program to calculate abovementioned parameters; discriminative functions were calculated with the help of step by step discriminative analysis in «SPSS Statistics 17.0» and «Statistica 6.0» programs.

Specificity implies the share of healthy people found healthy in the course of diagnostics from the total number of healthy.

Sensitivity implies the share of ill patients found ill in the course of diagnostics from the total number of ill patients.

Results and discussion

The first stage of the work consisted in step by step discriminative analysis including the control group and each of the three groups of arterial hypertension (according to degree of severity) separately. Results are presented in Table 1. The given figures are the result of cross-testing. The latter implies that each test is classified according to functions obtained in all test but the particular one.

Table 1. Grouping according to degree of AH. Results for all patients.

AH degree	specificity	sensitivity
AH1	67.6 %	62.0%
AH2	68.4%	66.5%
AH3	72.8%	77.9%

As an example we present discriminative function between the control group and the group of the 1st degree of AH severity. 8 parameters were included into the obtained discriminative function, among them were spectrum width of the images of the right thumb, sector of the head (cortex and vessels), suprarenals, thyroid and kidneys. Discriminative function for the control group and diagnosed AH1 group looks as follows:

$$D = 0.017*X_1+5.538*X_2-0.476*X_3+0.426*X_4+0.001*X_5- \\ +1.720*X_6+4.171*X_7+4.595*X_8-8.979$$

If X_1, X_2 etc are substituted in the course of the screening by values of measured parameters for the particular person, the tested patient either with 67.6% accuracy is being referred to the group of healthy, or with 62.0 % accuracy having the 1st degree of arterial hypertension and should undergo an additional testing.

From stage to stage of arterial hypertension the number of diagnostic parameters increases from 8 up to 19, which is understandable as it coincides which the degree of involvement of target-organs. All group proved to have the following sectors in common: cerebral cortex, thyroid and kidneys and starting with Group 2 (diagnosed AH2 of the 2nd degree) – the heart sector. Specificity and sensitivity increased along with higher degree of arterial hypertension.

It is known that GDV parameters are dependent of the patient's gender and arterial hypertension takes a different course in males and females [Hossu, Rupert 2006; Cohly et al 2009]. Discriminative functions were calculated for all three degrees of arterial hypertension for males and females separately (Table 2).

Table 2. Grouping according to AH degree. Results for males and females.

AH degree	Females		Males	
	Specificity	Sensitivity	Specificity	Sensitivity
AH1	76.4%	77.8%	80.9%	73.7%
AH2	74.2%	81.3%	63.8%	70.8%
AH3	75.3%	74.7%	78.7%	80.2%

Common diagnostic parameters were found for all groups, they included sectors of the cerebral cortex, vascular system, heart, thyroid and kidneys. Specificity and sensitivity of the functions obtained in groups divided on the basis of patients' gender were 5-9 % higher than for the mixed group.

The number of diagnostic parameters used and percentage of difference for females with AH1 and AH2 were found higher than that for males. Men are known to have a tendency for higher arterial pressure against women of reproductive age. Differences on AP between men and women disappear after women's menopause or ovarioectomy. AH incidence is lower in women below 60 and higher over 60 against men of similar age.

The next stage of the investigation was comparison of data obtained for patients of the control group and groups with different stages of arterial hypertension.

Specificity and sensitivity values of calculated discriminative functions increased from the first stage of arterial hypertension to the third. Increase in specificity from stage to stage amounted to 67-80 %, and sensitivity – to 70-77%. The number of diagnostic parameters increased from stage 1 to stage 3 from 7 to 22. For all stages sectors of the cerebral cortex, heart, suprarenals and thyroid were involved in calculation.

Table 3. Grouping according to AH stages. Results for the whole group.

AH stage	Specificity	Sensitivity
AHs1	66.9 %	70.9%
AHs2	67.6%	73.5%
AHs3	80.1%	76.5%

Discriminative functions were also calculated for men and women separately (Table 4).

Table 4. Grouping according to AH stages. Results for males and females.

AH stage	females		Males	
	Specificity	Sensitivity	Specificity	Sensitivity
AHs1	80.9%	64.1%	80.9%	79.5%
AHs2	68.1%	81.3%	75.3%	75.8%
AHs3	72.3%	67.3%	83.1%	84.4%

For this classification mean percentage of correct placements for men exceeded the one for women by 6-8%. It is likely to be associated with specific involvement of target organs for men and women.

Arterial hypertension is one of the main risk factors of cardiovascular diseases in women. Though the level of arterial pressure for women of the premenopause period is lower than for men of the corresponding age, AH incidence for elderly women is higher.

Discriminative functions were calculated to detect patients with different risk of cardio-vascular complications after arterial hypertension. Specificity and sensitivity of calculated functions amounted to 64% – 73.5% and 62.2% – 76% respectively which correlates with values for the groups classified on the basis of AH degree of severity. The number of diagnostic parameters increased depending on the risk group. Sectors reflecting the heart and kidneys were found as the most common for all groups (Tables 5,6).

Table 5. Grouping according to the risk of cardio-vascular complications. Results for the mixed group.

Risk of cardio-vascular complications	Specificity	Sensitivity
Risk 1	73.5 %	62.5%
Risk 2	69.9%	72.7%
Risk 3	64.0%	64.0%
Risk 4	69.9%	76.1%

Table 6. Grouping according to the risk of cardio-vascular complications.

Risk	Females		Males	
	Specificity	Sensitivity	Specificity	Sensitivity
Risk 1	82.0%	75.0%	76.6%	58.3%
Risk 2	78.7%	74.5%	70.2%	66.7%
Risk 3	74.2%	77.8%	74.5%	78.4%
Risk 4	76.4%	75.8%	68.1%	72.7%

Feasibility of detecting patients with different AH degrees was tested with the help of logistic regression. Specificity and sensitivity were found close in values to those obtained by discriminative analysis but values of specificity calculated by logistic regression were somewhat lower than those calculated by discriminative analysis which determined our choice of the latter in our investigations (Table 7).

Table 7. Grouping according to AH degrees. Results calculated by logistic regression.

AH degree	specificity	sensitivity
AH1	79.4 %	70.6%
AH2	68.3%	61.0%
AH3	58.1%	83.7%

Our findings correlate well with those obtained earlier by other investigators with the help of neuron network method as well as during comparison of the diagnosis made with the help of GDV and other diagnostic methods widely used in modern medicine [Stockley, Spiwak 2009].

Conclusions

Sectors of cerebral cortex, heart, thyroid, suprarenals and kidneys proved to be the most frequent diagnostic parameters. We believe that patients' grouping was most qualitative under classification according to AH stages, which may be explained by the fact that in grouping according to AH stages both degree of arterial pressure elevation and involvement of target organs were taken into account. Classification according to patients' gender increased the accuracy of diagnostics by 5-9% which was due to differences in development and course of arterial hypertension in women and men.

Thus, reliable differences between the control group of healthy patients and groups with various AH degrees and stages were calculated with sufficiently high degree of accuracy which allows to include Electrophotonic - Gas Discharge Visualization technique into the population screening.

Detection of Hidden Food Allergens

Well-known approach developed by Dr Voll of detection human reaction to different products by measuring acupuncture points while a person holds a product in a hand. Similar method was offered with GDV technique which is illustrated by the work of Volkov et al [2010].

Haemodiagnostics is a method of detecting hidden food allergens and choosing a diet for people with various illnesses has been tested over the years and has proved to be highly effective in outpatient clinical practice in the clinic of Dr Volkov. Haemodiagnostics of food was carried out by comparing the data of the obtained from Erythrocyte Segmentation Rate reaction (ESR) of blood with the addition of food extracts with the control (ESR blood without the addition of extract).

A volunteer with health problems was selected as a subject. GDV diagnostics of the same products (extracts) in the test tube which the subject held in his left hand, was performed as follows: changes in the GDV parameters of fingers of his right hand were compared with the control GDV parameters of the same finger when there was no tube in the left hand.The session consisted of taking pictures of 10 products and 10 controls.

Table. Indices of bioobject reaction to food *

Cabbage	Apple	Chicken	Millet	Mustard	Potatoes	Onions	Grapefruit
+2↑	+0,5↓	0≈	**+2↑**	**-1↓**	**-1↓**	+0,5↑	**+2↑**
-0,3	+15.3	+4,5	**+7,0**	**-0,1**	**-4,1**	-0.3	**+6,0**

* Deviations from the control in conditional relative units. Arrows indicate the direction of the deviation of index compared to the previous one.
First row – blood test; second row – GDV test.

The table shows haemodiagnostics data - deviations from the target ESR control for a number of products (their extracts). Clearly visible is a positive reaction of the blood to cabbage, millet, and grapefruit and negative to mustard and potatoes. This correlates with GDV data except cabbage. The level of correlation of GDV parameters with data of the ESR method indicates the prospects of further studies of the influence of various biological and synthetic liquid and solid substrates on man using this technique.

Part III. MONITORING OF PATIENTS' CONDITION AFTER DIFFERENT INFLUENCES

One of the advantages of Electrophotonic technique is its sensitivity to people emotional and physiological condition and its transformation under the influence of different stimulus. A lot of professionals use Electrophotonic in everyday practice and some of them present their findings at different conferences, in particular, at the annual Saint Petersburg Congress "Science, Information and Spirit". Below we shortly reference some of the known to us papers.

Hydrogen Peroxide Treatment

The patented method of treatment and prevention of the immunodeficiency (and therefore energy deficiency) organism's state is the inhalation (aerosol) therapy of the aqueous solution of the 0.01-1.5% hydrogen peroxide. Patients received the inhalation therapy in weekly courses of 5-30 minutes during 1-6 months. At the beginning of the procedures the hydrogen peroxide concentration was set to the most comfortable level for the patient and was increased by 0.01% after each course up to the maximal endurable dose. GDV technique was used to monitor condition of almost 1500 patients [Volkov et al 2005]. The main discovered features after the course were the following:

1. The image area visibly increased in the GDV-grams taken with filter, the integral area indices reached or exceeded their maximal values.
2. The energy deficient local zones disappeared or decreased in the "without filter" mode.
3. The area characteristics of the images were equalized in both registration modes.
4. The asymmetry of the images that was present before the introduction of the hydrogen peroxide was reduced, mainly in the registration mode without filter.
5. The diagram image was approaching a regular circle.

The GDV-grams were digitally processed and the following image characteristics were chosen as the GDV-parameters for investigation:

- Average (for all fingers) values of the following 10 parameters: glow area, form coefficient, average isoline radius, mean-square deviation (MSD) of the isoline radius from the finger average value, isoline length, entropy along the isoline, average intensity, number of fragments, fractality along the isoline, MSD of the fractality from the finger average value;
- MSD of the values of these parameters for individual fingers from the averages on all the fingers.

Statistical processing of data for different groups of patients are presented in Table and on the graph.

Table 1. The GDV-parameters that demonstrated significant difference in the "before the procedure (v)" and "after the procedure (V)" dependent samplings measured in the endocrine-diseases and musculoskeletal diseases groups without filter.

GDV-parameter	v < V, %	p-level (sign test)	p-level (Wilcoxon test)
Area	94	**0.001**	**0.001**
Average radius	75	*0.080*	**0.004**
Radius std	13	**0.006**	**0.001**
Isoline length	69	*0.211*	**0.015**
Entropy	88	**0.006**	**0.001**
Number of fragments	13	**0.006**	**0.001**
Intensity std	31	*0.211*	**0.034**

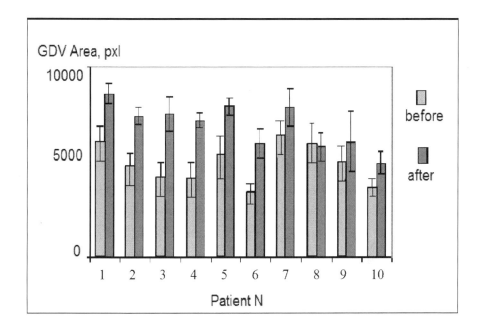

Fig. The Average Glow Area parameter values in the musculoskeletal-diseases group before and after the treatment procedure. The intervals on the diagram columns show the limits of the mean-square deviation (on 10 fingers) from the average value.

Presented data demonstrate efficiency of the GDV technique for monitoring patients' condition in the course of treatment.

Similar approach was applied in the work of Mercier Béatrice and Prost Josiane [2011] from Holiste Laboratory Le Port and Burgundy University Dijon. They evaluated the impact of Bol D'air Jacquier® Breathing Session on Human Energy Fields for 7 people. Authors carefully checked all GDV parameters and found significant effects both with and without filter. This is an example of case study, as they did not have neither control group, nor blind placebo testing. We are not sure to which level the effect of treatment was related to emotional responses.

Acupuncture Treatment

Interesting research on the evaluation of the effects of acupuncture treatment was done under supervision of Dr. Norm Shealy and Dr Willam Tiller [Rizzo-Roberts, 2004]. In this study, 33 randomly-chosen, clinically healthy subjects were utilized in a self- control fashion. Data from MSA-21 and GDV devices were gathered before and after double-blind needling at both true and sham acupuncture points. The study required two visits by each subject for needling at five different acupuncture points, one for true and one for sham needling. Indeed, the GDV instrument passed this test with flying colors and provided much useful adjunct information as well. Both of the MSA-21 and the GDV devices, as seen by the results of this study, can be used to conduct a comprehensive meridian stress assessment and to determine appropriate ways to achieve healthy energetic balance. The GDV instrument was able to distinguish authentic acupuncture needling from sham acupuncture needling. For healthy subjects, the GDV instrument detected a larger response to authentic needling compared to sham needling on the right side of the body relative to the left. This body asymmetry effect could be related to the direction of Qi-flow through the body and the relationship between the mental physical manifestation through the right and left hands.

The objective of the research by [Haydon 2005] was to detect any change in the human energy field of the body after the stimulation of Dr. Shealy's Rings of Fire, Earth, Water, Air, and Crystal. A control group of sham, non-acupuncture points was also administered. The acupuncture points were stimulated electrically using the SheLi Tens Stimulator. Dr. Shealy discovered and defined the naturally existing circuits with specific acupuncture points and named these circuits after the five basic elements of fire, air, water, earth, and crystal. Each ring is comprised of 12 to 13 points. Through his research Dr. Shealy has shown statistically significant results utilizing the acupuncture points in his rings [Shealy 2004]. 80 clinically healthy individuals, ranging from age 21 to 80 years of age were available for testing. 60 of the participants were in the age range of 45 to 65; however, there were a few subjects in the twenties, thirties, seventies, and eighties. 33 of the volunteers were male and 57 were female. Not all of the subjects completed the whole set of six tests. 61 participants completed the Ring of Fire and control test. 59 participants completed Ring of Water. 57 completed Ring of Earth. 56 completed the Ring of Air, and 55 participants completed the Ring of Crystal. Over 30 subjects completed the whole set of the five rings and a set of sham points.

Results of statistical analysis averaged on the group are presented in the Table.

Table. An overview of the data analysis in the paired t-test.

	Left hand Without filter	Right hand Without filter	Left hand With filter	Right hand With filter
Ring of Water	Yes $p<.05$	Yes $p<.001$	No	No
Ring of Fire	No	No	No	No
Ring of Crystal	Yes $p<.05$	Yes $p<.01$	Yes $p=.05$	No
Ring of Earth	Yes $p<.001$	Yes $p<.05$	No	Yes $p<.01$
Ring of Air	Yes $p<.001$	Yes $<.001$	No	No
Control	No	No	No	No

In the Ring of Fire, there was no statistically significant change ($p<.05$) with or without a filter in the readings before and after stimulation of the *average* value as shown in the paired t-test. However, detailed analysis of data shows that stimulation of this ring creates the most significant change when compared to all the other rings. This is due to the "balance point" being right in the middle of the sample, where half of the people went up in JS value and the other half went down, thus canceling any change on the average JS value. This concurs with Dr. Shealy's research which indicates that the Ring of Fire is the most important ring, as it raises DHEA to a normal level in the body.

Participants in the study, across all conditions (i.e., pretest, posttest, control, all six rings, each hand, and each filter setting) demonstrated extraordinary consistency in their energy readings, with nearly all JS readings falling within the normal range (i.e., -0.6 to +1.0). Clearly, this data set, drawn as it was from very healthy persons, is characterized by the statistical condition known as 'restriction of range.' That is, there is so little variability in the range of energy readings that any significant changes from pre- to posttest, or any significant differences between left and right hands are essentially precluded.

However, high and low levels of energy mean different things for different individuals. Just like a headache has a multitude of meanings as a symptom, low or high energy in the body can mean many things. The energy field is constantly in motion and many readings over different times are needed to determine any consistency of the pattern for each individual.

While the initial approach focused on the change of the average JS value, the final analysis showed that the most significant effect for all rings except the Ring of Crystal was a movement of the reading toward what we have defined as a balance point. So on average, those who started out above this JS value were pulled down toward it, and those who started out below this value were pulled up toward it. For the Ring of Crystal all subjects were pulled up in JS value on average. All the other rings were stimulating the body for a specific chemical or hormone, whereas the Ring of Crystal was removing free radicals from the body. Therefore, the most significant result of this study was this movement toward homeostasis in the body for all rings, not just an overall increase or decrease in average value as was initially thought.

Author concludes as follows: "The GDV camera can be an excellent biofeedback tool. The volunteers revealed it in the interaction and responses. Everyone wanted copies of the testing and was anticipating the change in his before and after graphs. This suggests that, if one physically sees the feedback, he may be able to create a lifestyle that contributes to better mental and physical health. It might also enhance better health to see the change before and after such activities as hypnotherapy, exercise, or massage therapy".

In the work [Lyapko et al 2006] 38 patients suffering from wound dystrophy of spinal cord, 27 men and 11 women, age from 19 to 52 years old, had treatment course at Burdenko Sanatorium in the City of Saki, Crimea. All patients were divided into two groups. The first group included 16 persons who had the course of standard treatment including electric stimulation and mud cure. The second group consisted of 22 patients who were given, additionally to standard treatment, the full course of 10 applications therapy using various metals multi-needle applicators developed by Doctor N. Lyapko. Analysis of patients with GDV technique demonstrated statistical difference of GDV indexes both averaged between groups, and for every patient in experimental group between initial and after treatment readings.

The results of investigation demonstrate that data dynamics in the both groups reflects the reaction development stages of organism to the course of treatment: initially the energy increase of blood circulation system was detected accompanied with the tendency to endocrine system (zone of epiphysis) activation. In next days the reaction of endocrine system and small bowels got of paramount importance. During the last group of GDV graphic study the reaction of backbone (sacral bone) was the mostly expressed one, as well as that of heart while it was not so expressed with kidneys. It worth mentioning that all changes were expressed with data picked up from the left hand fingers.

Comparing the data between the groups we got reliable differences in the energy of small, ascending and end part of large bowels, as well as in the liver zone, lymphatic and endocrine systems, coronary blood vessels and spinal column. Besides, the differences between the right-side and left-side energy (unbalance) got reliable.

Course of Systemic Medicine by Jose Olaldo

Systemic Medicine is effective mechanism developed in Venezuela by Jose Olalde and his team to fight the consequences of chronic degenerative diseases, having demonstrated in a short time its capacity to soothe and solve many pathologies [Olalde 2003-2005]. In the course of treatment doctors are using specially selected natural adaptogens which was shown to be efficient in many chronic situations. A Retrospective, Multicentric, and Comparative Study was undertaken, based on data collected in the Adaptogene Medical Educational Centers (CMA) at La Trinidad and Sabana Grande. Subjects of the study was 119 patients who suffered chronic sicknesses, of an age between 7 and 90 years -average of 57.6 years- 65 were females (54.6%) and 54 were males (45.3%). Patients were evaluated with GDV instrument initially and several time in the course of treatment. The bioelectric field, at each evaluation, was higher than the one at the initial examination. At the second medical evaluation, the average increase was +27,7% compared with the initial examination. At the third medical evaluation, an average increase of +26% was observed, compared with the initial examination. Finally, at the fourth evaluation, the increase was +28,4% compared with the initial examination.

ANALYSIS OF PATIENTS WITH ARTERIAL HYPERTENSION (AH)

Of the 40 cases of AH reported at the beginning of the study, 12 of them suffered from arterial hypertension controlled with synthetic drugs, and therefore were excluded from the analysis. The uncontrolled Average Arterial Tension (A.A.T.) of 28 patients with AH was calculated, assessing the values obtained from A.A.T. differences, before and after Systemic Medicine treatment. The clinical reply to A.A.T. treatment with Systemic Medicine was demonstrated, and at the same time the functional energy reserves increased.

ANALYSIS OF PATIENTS WITH DIABETES TYPE 2

A sample of 10 patients with diabetes type 2 was taken. Their glycemia values before and after -Systemic Medicine treatment- were determined. They showed an improvement in their energy levels (area GDV) and a reduction of glycemia levels.

DIABETIC FOOT AMPUTATION RISK

A retrospective cohort study was carried out in 98 patients with diabetic foot grades D1-D3. Patients were treated with a standardized systemic plant extract combination -Circulat- in combination with conventional therapy. Electrophotonics Area and Activation Index were evaluated before and after treatment. A correlation was confirmed between patients' clinical improvement and alterations in Electrophotonic (Ep) measurements. Circulat prevented 88.5% of amputations, a figure which is higher than conventional treatments and normalized the Area and Activation Index values in 97.56% and 95.12% of the patients respectively. Although the number of patients who's, after treatment, Electrophotonic's Activation Index and Area values remained outside of the normal values was very small, it is worth noting that all of them had amputations. The after treatment probability of amputation in diabetic foot patients with normal values in Area and Activation Index was very low: 8.33% and 6.38%, respectively. Normalizing the Area and Activation Index values -with a reliable treatment, such as Circulat in conjunction with conventional therapy- diminished the amputation risk.

VARIATION IN QUALITY OF LIFE (QOL)

The parameter Quality of Life improved in 94,5% of the patients at the second evaluation, with an average variation of 13,01%. At the third evaluation, 98% of the patients increased their QoL -compared with the initial evaluation- with a 21% variation. At the fourth evaluation, 100% of the patients assessed enhanced their QoL with an average variation of 34%. The average value of QoL of the patients was, at the beginning of the treatment, 74,28%. This developed to reach an average value of 88,8% at the last evaluation which was an average increase of 19,6% compared with the initial value.

It has been shown that a low level of functional energy reserves corresponds to a chronic pathology and that a clinical improvement of the patient with Systemic Medicine was related with an increase of the total area of the bioelectric field. From this we can infer that the functional energy reserve is an important indicator of the general condition of the patient. In effect, there exists a correlation between the variation of the GDV image and the clinical evolution of the patient whose functional energy reserves are affected. The normalization in the area corresponds to an improvement of the clinical manifestations of patients with chronic diseases.

Light Therapy

In Federal State Institution "Dzerzhinsky Central Clinical Sanatorium of Federal Security Service of the Russian Federation" the research was carried out with 56 children from 6 to 9 years old (average age was 6.6±1.8 years), staying at sanatorium under treatment for 21 days, with respiratory system diseases: chronic diseases of tonsils and adenoids (34 people), chronic rhinopharyngitis (18 people), lower air passages - recurrent bronchitis (4 people) [Bykov et al 2006]. All children received traditional therapies of sanatorium-and-spa treatment: climatotherapy, including sea- and pool-bathing, exercise therapy, balneotherapy, hydrotherapy, physiotherapy (phytoinhalations, UV-radiation treatment of nasal and fauces cavities).

In addition the experimental group (28 children) – besides traditional sanatorium-and-spa therapy, underwent infra-red laser therapy on wings of nose, on projection of nasopharynx, maxillary sinuses and submaxillary lymph nodes combined with laser reflexotherapy according to contact methods with exposition of 1-2 minutes per area. The total course of treatment made up 10 procedures. Besides that, over-venous blood exposure (ulnar vein) using reflecting nozzle was held every other day. The course made up 5 procedures.

Both groups were equal in age, nosology and were different only in using the course of laser therapy.

$\frac{35}{17}$ The analysis of personal complaints and data of objective research are evidence of positive dynamics in both groups, however more distinct dynamics can be noticed in the second group.

$\frac{35}{17}$ The analysis of figures of cardiointervalogram is the evidence of the following:

Ĥ   the main group is notable for: increasing of total intensity of neurohumoral modulation (86% of patients – 24 people); 14% of patients – 4 people – didn't show distinct dynamics of that parameter. 82% of patients (23 people) showed the tendency for equilibration of vegetative modulation of heart rate at primary checked measurements, which could be characterized by excessive activation of parasympathetic part of vegetative nervous system.

Ĥ   the control group is notable for: increasing of total intensity of neurohumoral modulation (65% of patients – 18 people); decreasing of total intensity of spectre, expressed by certain degree. 50% of patients (14 people) showed the tendency for equilibration of vegetative modulation of heart rate at primary excessive activation of parasympathetic part of vegetative nervous system

Ĥ   The analysis of common non-specific adaptive response:

Ĥ   the transfer from reaction of tranquil activation to reaction of increased activation was discovered at 78% patients from the first group (22 people) and at 50% from the second group (14 people), and that is the evidence of positive dynamics. Other examined patients from main and control groups didn't have certain modified figures of leukogram.

Ĥ Results of GDV analysis: the improvement of GDV-gram indices for both groups: certain increasing of area and density of luminescent glow, the infill of faulty areas, while this effect was more pronounced in the experimental group.

Ĥ 62% of patients of the experimental group demonstrated significant improvement of GDV indexes:

GDV Index	Before treatment	After treatment
The integral glow square (S-integ)	Right - 0.39±0.61	0.026±0.47
S-integ	Left - 0.41±0.78	0.003±0.39
Hypophysis area	Right 0.41±0.28	0.54±0.39
Hypothalamus area	Right - 0.53±0.27	- 0.09±0.21
Coronary vessels	Right 0.12±0.36	0.57±0.27
Coronary vessels	Left 0.02±0.44	0.46±0.38
Urinary system	Right - 1.26±0.38	-0.19±0.41

All changes before – after were statistically significant with $p < 0.01$

Ĥ In control group 54% of patients demonstrated significant increase of GDV index S-integ ($p<0.01$).

Increase of sectional area in endocrine system areas (hypophysis, hypothalamus), coronary vessels and urinary system was expressed less in comparison with the experimental group.

The effect of light therapy with BIOCOM-LUX system was studied by Eusebio González Martín from Spain [Martin 2011]. This system emits light into Violet part of spectrum (390-410 nm). Based on population of 25 people author has demonstrated significant effect of Energy Field transformation after the treatment.

Music Therapy

Music is a great achievement of our Civilization. Billions of people do not imagine their life without music, and there are a lot of approaches to use music as a part of healing process.

In experiments conducted by Kalashnikova E.O. et al [2001] effect of music therapy was tested on a group of 20 drug-addicted juvenile delinquents aged 16-21. During the courses (7-10 courses per month, 40 minutes each) the teenagers were listening to the audio recordings of Russian spiritual music, chime and classic music (organ, harp, lute). GDV-grams were taken before and after a course. Besides, the psychological test according to Lucher was used.

Results demonstrated gradual improvement of GDV-parameters (for 30% on average) with each course. After the third course the GDV-parameters were stabilizing. The psychological test revealed a lower level of anxiousness among 80% of the teenagers (in 1.8-2.1 times), 90% of the tested became less aggressive, fractious and irascible. We could also observe higher workability. The intensified activity of sympathetic nervous system was registered among 90% of the teenagers. Moreover, the individuals suffering from phobias normalized their night sleep (quicker falling asleep and a less number of spontaneous awakening). Those who suffered from tic recovered. We could also observe improvement of memory.

Gibson S. and Williams B. [2005] studied the effect of music and focused meditation on the human energy field and profile of mood states. 49 subjects participated; mean age 50.47+/-25; 7 men and 42 women; 19 were healthy, with no diagnosis and no medication and 30 subjects had a variety of diagnoses including depression, ADD, arthritis, breast cancer, diabetes fibromyalgia, gerd, glaucoma, heart condition, high cholesterol, Lymphodema, multiple sclerosis, osteoporosis, Parkinson's. People listened to music of the Baroque period, a Pachelbel Canon in D for 15 minutes.

There were statistically significant improvements on the POMS-Total score, POMS-Tension and POMS-Depression scores decreased by 7.00 and 6.25 points respectively, p< 0.001. There was also a statistically significant 1.68 drop in the Subjective Units of Distress (SUDS) scale after the music intervention, p<. 001, moving from stressed to calm.

For GDV Area and GDV Br, t-test results indicated a statistically significant increase in both parameters: GDV Area t (47)=2.725, p < 0.01, and GDV Br (47)=4.391, p < 0.001, i.e. the energy field grew larger and brighter. Tests indicated a significant result for GDV-Anxiety, z=2.19, p<0.05.

The influence of music was tested in Medical Academy of Spiritual Development "MADRA" together with Lugansk state medical university (Ukraine) [Semenichin et al 2011]. Over a period of 3 years the total of 120 persons was subjected to musictherapy sessions and have been examined with EPI technique. Classical music of various composers – I.S.Bach, L.V. Beethoven, S.Rahmaninov, P.I.Tchaikovsky, A.Prokofiev, V.A.Mozart, A.Vivaldi, etc. - has been used.

As a result of investigation it has been established that after listening to music the change of energy and improvement of psycho-emotional status of patients were noted. For example, listening to Symphony №6 by P.I.Tchaikovsky 53.8% of patients showed reliable increasing of total area of luminescence and harmonization of an energy field. Symphony №40 by V.A.Mozart - showed 33.3%. Symphony №5 by L.V. Beethoven - 58.3% of patients. Listening Concert for the piano with an orchestra №1 by P.I.Tchaikovsky 46.7% of cases showed increasing. 46.7% of cases showed decreasing of a total area of luminescence. Listening to Brandenburg concert №1 by I.S.Bach the total area of luminescence showed increase to 42.9%. decrease to 14.3% of patients. and no change in 42.8%.

The assessment of individual sensitivity to various music was the next task. For example, volunteer K. in the given experiment showed increase of luminescence area at listening to Concert for the piano with an orchestra №2 by S.Rahmaninov by 4.9% (reduction of entropy by 2.0%). to Symphony №5 by L.V. Beethoven - 11.2% (entropy was increased by 6.5%). to Symphony №6 by P.I.Tchaikovsky - 5.7% (increase of entropy by 11.0%). However, organ mass by I.S.Bach led to

81

potential decrease by 2.9% (reduction of entropy by 1.4%). Thus it has been established that music effect on an individual and music of various composers unequally influence GDV indicators of the same person.

During the experiment various effects on body organs and systems have been observed. For example, listening to Concert for the piano with an orchestra №2 by S.Rahmaninov showed reliable increasing of luminescence area in sectors of hypothalamo-pituitary-adrenal system in more than 60% of cases, the increasing in sector of coronary vessels and respiratory system was also observed. At the same time effect of Brandenburg concert №1 by I.S.Bach was observed in sectors characterizing vessels of a brain (the increasing of luminescence area has been noted in 71.4% of cases, reduction - in 21.4%), coronary vessels (in 50% and 7,1% of cases, accordingly), the nervous system (28.6% and 57.1%).

The luminescence area and entropy have proved the most informative indicators in GDV-image analysis after music therapy. The luminescence area and entropy change is in various degrees sometimes unidirectional, and sometimes differently directed, which complicates individual selection of music.

For a complex assessment of effect of music on energy status of a person the vibratory coefficient which is defined on the basis of value of luminescence area and entropy was offered. The vibratory coefficient reflects system character of music effect on a human body and its psycho-emotional status. Increasing of this coefficient for the person after listening to music is indicated by a larger degree of music corresponding to a vibratory key of the person. In this research the increasing of coefficient by 3 ... 30%, in case when music fitted a certain person was observed. Decreasing of vibratory coefficient indicates that the given music does not fit the person.

For example, in patient B at listening to organ mass by I.S.Bach the vibratory coefficient was increased by 10.7%; to Concert for the piano with an orchestra №1 by P.I.Tchaikovsky by 8.2%. Symphony №40 by V.A.Mozart by 3.1% which allows to recommend the given music to this person. But listening to Symphony №5 by L.V. Beethoven and Symphony № 6 by P.I.Tchaikovsky led to coefficient decreasing by 5.3% (fig. 3).

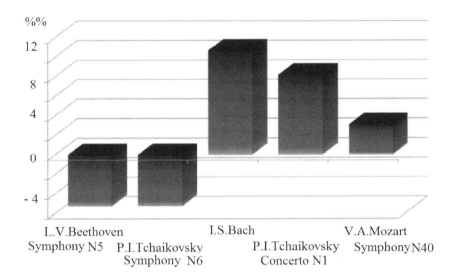

Fig. Change of vibratory coefficient for a person after listening music

Noted essential changes of luminescence in various people at listening to the same music testify to necessity of individual selection of music. It may help people return the lost harmony of the soul with world around, as macrocosm and microcosm work under the eternal law of music - the harmony law.

The Effect of Different Trainings

The subjects of this study [Cowan 2006] included two groups: N=41 who received Crystal Bowl treatment as the independent variable and N=41 the control group who did not receive treatment. In the treatment group, the Crystal Bowl was set to the tone of C. Each subject received fifteen minutes of either Crystal Bowl toning or Control group sitting quietly. 86 participants were recruited for this study, ages 18 through 79. A total of 82 subjects completed the study. The treatment and control group completed the pre-POMS questionnaires, three baseline GDV readings, five minutes apart. This was followed after five minutes a post-GDV reading, completion of the post-POM including a twenty minute period followed by a final post GDV reading.

First, it was important to examine the stability of the baseline measures in both the treatment and control groups across the seven chakras comparing baselines utilizing correlation coefficients. Cross comparisons were calculated among all three baselines measures within each subject. This comparison shows very stable data with an average correlation value of $r = 0.735$ $p<0.01$. In both treatment and control groups only a few outlying individuals did not have stable baselines, as shown, in Fig., which plots the ranked correlations between baselines measures 2 and 3.

Next figure shows the average control group reading vs. the average treatment group reading after the experiment. The graph clearly demonstrates a response in the first, fifth and seventh chakra, however, only the fifth chakra difference is statistically significant ($p = 0.001$). In this study what we were really attempting to demonstrate is any response, either positively or negatively (-6.0 to +6.0) to the sound of the crystal bowl on the chakas utilizing the GDV. Example of Pre and two Post GDV Readings for participant 01 from treatment group is given at fig. 3.

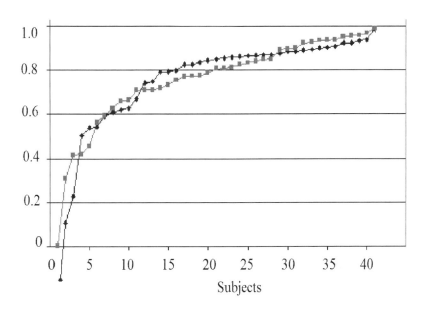

Fig. Stability of the Baselines: scatter plot between baselines 2 and 3 for treatment and control groups.

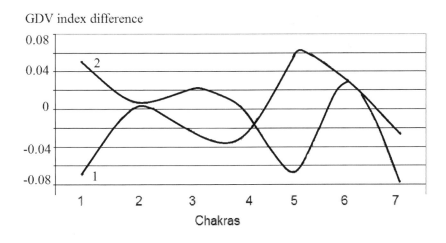

Fig . Average pre-post difference of GDV readings Across 7 Chakras for Treatment (2) and Control (1) groups

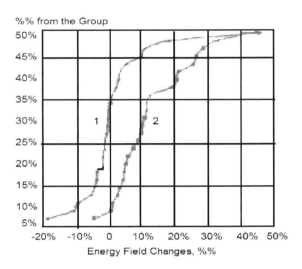

Fig. Energy response of people to EMF Balancing Technique training in Germany (1) and USA (2) [Lutz Rabe, 2009].

In the work of Lutz Rabe [2009] from the Institute for Bioelectrophotonics Germany studies on the effect of personal development training for the Phase 9-12 of the EMF Balancing Technique training classes were performed during training in the USA and Germany. Analysis of GDV data demonstrated very similar distribution of human reactions in both cases, but in Germany response was stronger (curve 1 on the graph).

From other research lines we should mention paper presented by Korotkov K, Bundzen P, Bronnikov V and Lognikova L. in 2005 on Bioelectrographic correlates of the direct vision phenomenon – Russian training of children to read texts and operate in space without using their eyes.

Dr Samuel A. Berne studies the effect of dolphins on the human biofield using GDV analysis [Berne 2011]. People were measured before and after swimming with dolphins. The average person's biofield was becoming more coherent and compressed, leading to a better health and wellness.

For many years research of human response to different exercises with EPI technique was conducted by Paul Dobson and Elena O'Keeffe from City University, London [Dobson 2000, 2005, 2012].

This was an empirical study of the relationships between photon emission as measured by the GDV technique and the "Big Five" personality dimensions as measured by NEO-FFI. Samples in Russia (N = 35) and the UK (N = 42) completed the NEO-FFI and the GDV procedure administered by a trained GDV operator. A strong relationship (R = .69, p < .000) was found between the extent of photon emission as measured by GDV parameters and one of the "Big Five" personality dimensions, namely, Openness to Experience. This relationship held for both sub-samples when analyzed separately (UK, R = .60, p < .002; Russian, R = .53, p < .015) and for all the fingers of both hands. The research also found some significant results for Extraversion but these were not as strong or as consistent as those for Openness. Insignificant results were found for the other three personality dimensions measured by the NEO, namely, Neuroticism, Agreeableness and Conscientiousness.

IN a later study a wide range of interventions each led by an experienced tutor were included in the research: T'ai Chi; Kundalini Yoga; Meditation; Healing by a Tibetan lama; The Progressive Muscle Relaxation; Stress Management Training; The Unwinding group chose their usual day-to-day method of relaxation more or less equal measure, smoking, drinking or meditation. The total sample for the research therefore involved 82 reportedly stressed individuals distributed between 8 different types of intervention, and a "control" group of 15.

Table 1: Case-by-case analysis of the impact of stress intervention on GDV Area

	% Cases with statistically* significant increase in GDV finger images	% Cases with no change in GDV finger images	% Cases with statistically* significant decrease in GDV finger images
Meditation	66%	17%	17%
T'ai Chi	60%	30%	10%
Unwinding	57%	43%	0%
Muscle Relaxation	56%	44%	0%
Acupuncture	56%	33%	11%

Stress Workshop	50%	30%	20%
T'ai Chi (HIV)	40%	60%	0%
Tibetan Healing	33%	56%	11%
Kundalini Yoga	20%	53%	27%
Control Group	25%	62.5%	12.5%

*probability of the change occurring by chance is less than 0.05.

The results show that the GDV image of most participants increased during the majority of the interventions designed to reduce stress. In many cases this was very visible and dramatic. As the table above indicates, highly significant subject differences were found. That is, the same intervention affects different people differently. For example, meditation appears to have a positive benefit for the majority, but no effect or a negative impact for others. Authors concluded that whilst you cannot tell whether or not an individual *feels* stressed from their GDV images, an experienced reduction in reported stress levels is commonly associated with an increase in the GDV image area. This finding also emphasises the importance of investigating the GDV on a case-by-case basis.

The final stage in our analysis of the data involved an investigation to see whether there were any significant individual or finger differences in response to these various interventions. No significant finger differences were found. That is, regardless of whether the overall change in finger image area was positive or negative, the impact tended to affect all the fingers equally. This points to a general metabolic or biophysical response, rather than a specific response where different fingers or finger sectors reflect different body systems.

The overall conclusion by the authors was as follows: "So we reason that cognition and personality influence photon emission because they influence our physiological responses which in turn affect body capacitance. Perhaps the physiological reactions that result in the mobilisation of body energy are key, for example, those that affect blood sugar levels and ATP production, but there may be a bundle of responses having effects on capacitance. This rationale is able to explain why physical relaxation, meditation, calming music and alcohol (it counteracts the effects of adrenalin) result in an increase in GDV image area; they reduce arousal, promote energy storage and increase capacitance. And why mental work by students, modelling of emotions by actors and preparation for competition by athletes result in a decrease in image area; they increase arousal, mobilise body energy and reduce capacitance".

Energy Healing

Electrophotonic instrument is very efficient for monitoring effects of Energy Healing. Several papers were published documenting this process.

Beverly Rubik published several cases of changes occurring in the human energy pattern after a specific intervention or consciousness-altering activity [Rubik 2004]. Several people were measured before and after 30-minute standard treatment of Therapeutic Touch to a pain. The general expansion and greater smoothness of the aura, and the filling in of gaps or discontinuities, indicating improved energy regulation following the practice of Therapeutic Touch was noted.

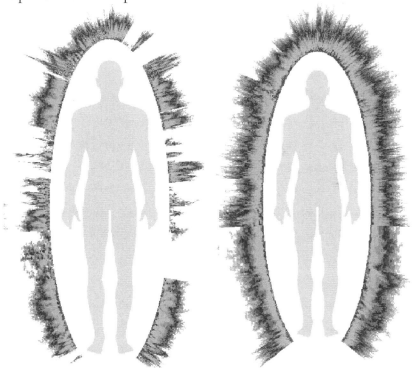

Fig. Energy Field of a person before and after Therapeutic Touch session.

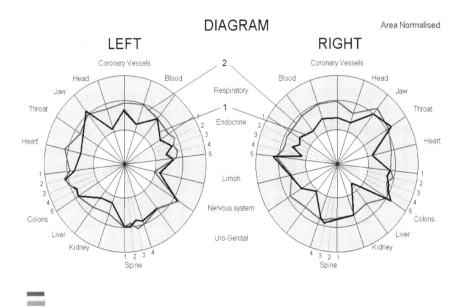

Fig. Energy diagram of a person before (1) and after (2) Therapeutic Touch session.

This was a preliminary experiment involving 2 subjects to see if the hypnotic command to "reduce energy" and produce glove anesthesia in the left hand would produce a corresponding measurable lateral change in the human energy pattern. Two professional hypnotists were employed as subjects, and each of them hypnotized the other sequentially. Relative energy distribution on the left and right sides of the body before and after hypnosis was calculated. The data show that before hypnosis, there was a small but insignificant difference in the energy on the right and left side of the body, with slightly more (0.023) on the left. However, upon hypnosis with an induction to create glove anesthesia in the left hand, significantly more energy appeared on the left side of the body with the less negative figure obtained (–0.312) compared to that on the right (–0.638). This result suggests that the process of hypnotic induction for glove anesthesia in the left hand involves entering into an altered state with expanded energy regionally specific in the body (in this case, left side). This finding is consistent with the fact that highly specific hypnotic inductions in hypnotizable subjects are known to create highly specific perceptions and behaviors in the subjects.

A group of people was studied before and after Practicing Dayan (Wild Goose) Qigong [Rubik 2005]. Effect of exercise was found different for different people.

A single-blind quasi-experimental study investigated the effect of remote intercessory prayer on several indicators of psychological and physical health and well-being was done by Janet Dunlop [2004]. GDV measures of psycho-physical condition; two self-assessment measures of health and well-being, the Profile of Mood States (POMS), and the Symptom Index (SI); and the levels of two hormones, DHEA and cortisol, and their ratio were used to assess changes. Participants were blind to their group assignment and were randomly selected across age groups (35 – 51, and above age 51) and three locations to either an IP group receiving remote intercessory prayer (n = 42), or a control group (n = 43).). Using a specific prayer, the investigator prayed non-locally for each IP participant, once weekly during the 12-week duration of the IP participant's study interval.

Discriminant function analysis (DFA) was used to predict group assignment (experimental or control) based on knowledge of the change scores for the GDV, the POMS, the SI and the intervening prayer beliefs. For the DFA, data were used from the 46 study participants who had complete data on all of the variables. All variables were entered into the equation at once, regardless of the individual difference in the groups. The model was significant in predicting group assignment (Wilks' lambda = . 37, χ^2 = 33.62, p = .029). The model correctly classified 91% of the total sample: 100% of the control group (n = 22) and 83% of the experimental group membership (n = 20 of 24). This classification difference could be explained by the greater within-group variance among the experimental group. The top five variables in descending order of significance were: posttest belief in the power of prayer for others (p = .01), posttest belief in prayer for self (p = .02), the GDV non-filter right hand area integer change score (p = .035), the non-filter right ring finger entropy change score (p = .06), and the stress index improvement value (p = .07). Thus, the DFA found one GDV measure--the non-filter right hand area integer--to be a significant predictor of group membership. In this study, the GDV appears to have been a much more sensitive measure than the POMS or the SI in detecting subtle, yet significant change from a prayer intervention.

For many years a healing society "Cosmo-Energy" founded by Emil Bagirov in Russia successfully organizes training and healing sessions for thousands of people. Since the end of 1990s a series of complex experiments have been regularly held during "Cosmo-Energy" sessions under the guidance of Professor of Physics, Victor Sharkov (Ph.D.). In the course of healing sessions a lot of unusual effects were recorded and documented, some of the results have been published in Russian and in [Sharkov, Bagirov 2011].

73 people were weighed before and after several healing sessions. Instrument: electronic scales, "Terraillon", BE-515G (error < 100 g).

1.1. In 85% of cases the change of weight was recorded, both decreasing and increasing, from 100 to 2000 g (from 3.5 to 70.5 oz) which constituted 0.15-3% of the weight of the participant.

1.2. Maximum changes of weight were recorded during first 20-40 min. of the session.

1.3. After the end of the session the weight returned to the background value within 15-30 min.

1.4. The weight changes' direction depended upon the emotional state of participants: positive emotions related to "Spiritual" aspects resulted in the decrees of weight, while negative emotions and memories resulted in the increase of weight; thoughts about everyday matters (work, home, children) in most cases had no effect on weight.

A series of radioactivity measurements during the healing sessions in 2005-2010 was performed. 30 min. after the beginning of the healing session the level of radiation typically dropped down by 30-60%. This level of radioactivity sustained during 30-40 min., and then returned to the background level. Simultaneous measurements outside the auditorium demonstrated no deviations from the basic level of radioactivity.

During a session the increase of infra-sound in the 4-8 Hz range by 2-5 decibel was recorded. This effect was repeated several times in the course of all sessions.

Large series of experiments was carried out measuring participants' Energy Field before and after healing sessions by means of GDV Electrophotonic instrument. In all cases the increase and harmonization of the Energy Field after healing sessions was recorded. For a group of 160 participants EPI parameters were calculated and this effect was found statistically significant for Energy Field and Intensity ($p < 0.05$).

During the 20th Annual ISSSEEM Conference in June 2010, many presentations were devoted to different modalities of healing. This topic is of importance both for the practice of CAM and for understanding the mechanisms of consciousness. In the scope of the conference a full-day workshop was presented; "Real-Time Measurements of the Human

Energy Field: Quantifying Subtle Energies with the Electrophotonic Imaging based on Gas Discharge Visualization Technique." During that workshop a series of experiments were conducted using Reconnective Healing, group intention, and a novel use of didgeridoo for sound therapy [Korotkov, De Vito et al 2010]. The EPC/GDV techniques show the effects of the healing and group intention activities. In addition, the ambient energetic activity of the workshop room was monitored during various eras, using the new antenna device that has been added to the Electrophotonic Imaging/Gas Discharge Visualization camera system. Interesting variation in the ambient energy was observed among the various eras with different workshop activities. Results presented in the paper are consistent with the previous observations that Reconnective Healing has significant effects for the energy state of the participants. Furthermore, data from the "Sputnik" sensor may be interpreted as transformations of the entropy of space, under the influence of the specific healing modality. The significant effects of water transformation under the influence of collective intention may be partly attributed to this factor as well.

During 2008-2010 several series of experiments during Reconnective Healing workshops and conferences in the USA and Europe have been performed. In all cases EPC instruments was used, in September 2008 three groups performed measurements in parallel: Ann Linda Baldwin and Gary E. Schwartz with heart rate variability and cutaneous blood perfusion techniques; William Tiller and Walter E. Dibble, with water Temperature and PH sensor; and Krishna Madappa and Konstantin Korotkov with EPC technology. All three groups independently recorded statistically significant effects of the Reconnective Healing with the participants. Results are presented in the book "Science Confirms Reconnective Healing" edited by K. Korotkov and available from Amazon.com.

Acclimatization to High Altitudes

The problem of acclimatization to high altitudes is important both for tourists visiting mountain areas and for people obliged to work at high elevation. A lot of research papers was dedicated to this problem and it si very important developing simple instrument to follow up acclimatization process.

In the work of [Bordes et al 2006] GDV readings were taken every night from a group of 8 people having trekking in Caucasus Mountains. On the 27.07 group arrived to the Caucasus Mountains and in two days people climbed two 4000 m peaks. On the 31.07 they moved to the hotel in the village Terscol at 2000 m. 01.08 group came to the slopes of Elbrus mountain and slept overnight at 3600 m. 02.08 people worked from 3600 m to 4200 m and after lunch came back to the hotel. 03.08 group moved to Ullu-tau area and for two nights camped there walking at day to different nearby places. 05.08 group came back to the hotel. For all participants a strong increase of Area and Intensity parameters at the Elbrus slopes (3600 m – 01.08) was found (see graphs). After descending to 2000 m (02.08) parameters dropped, but differently for different people. Strong increase in Area and Intensity was measured 03.08 and 04.08 at the Ullu-Tau mountains area and some decrease for most people 05.08.

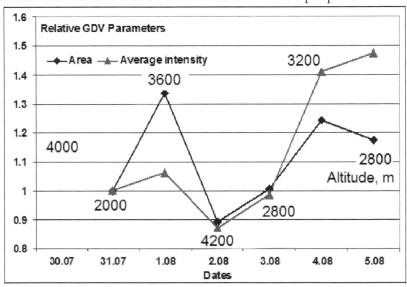

Fig. Time dynamics of GDV parameters during mountain trip.

94

As we see from these graphs, GVD parameters reflect the process of peoples' acclimatization to high altitudes.

In their next paper Sylvie Bordes discusses the application of nutrition for better acclimatization [Bordes 2011]. She gives detailed analysis of different supplement actions and propose recommendations for the optimal combination, The work is based on author's personal experience in many mountain expeditions and on the use of Electrophotonic analysis.

Process of acclimatization of Paralympic athletes of Russian national team was studied by [Drozdovski et al 2012]. Two EPI parameters were used for the study: Energy Potential, calculated from 0 to 100% and Stress Level, calculated from 0 to 10. Research was conducted for a team of 18 athletes in August 2011 and August 2012 in Bulgaria at the altitude 1820 m and in November 2011 and March 2012 in Switzerland at the altitude 2000 m. It was shown that these parameters reflect the level of individual acclimatization and help coacher to organize the process of preparation to the competitions.

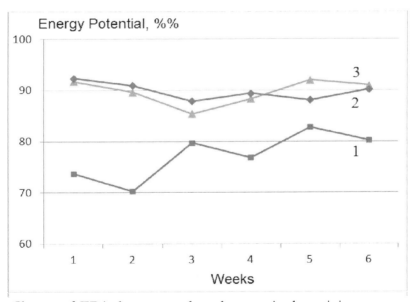

Fig. Change of EP index averaged on the team in the training camp.
1 - November 2011, Switzerland; 2 - March 2012 ,Switzerland; 3 - August 2012, Bulgaria. We may see that adaptation process to high altitudes being quite strong in 2011, resulted in fast acclimatization in 2012.

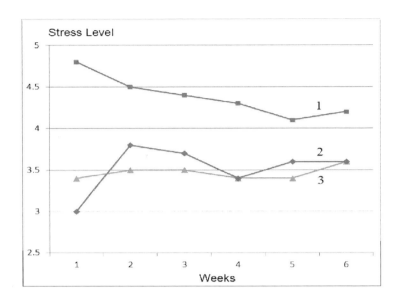

Fig. Change of Stress index averaged on the team in the training camp.
1 - November 2011, Switzerland; 2 – March 2012 ,Switzerland; 3 – August 2012, Bulgaria. We may see that adaptation process to high altitudes being quite strong in 2011, resulted in fast acclimatization in 2012.

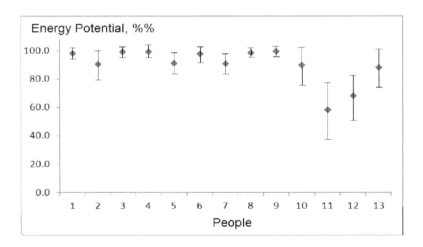

Fig, Average values and standard deviation of EP index for individual athletes in day-by-day measurements during training session in March 2012 in Switzerland at the altitude 2000 m. We may see difference between top-level athletes (N 1-9) and yang Paralympic athletes (N 10-13).

Response to Mobile Phone

The problem of the influence of mobile phones radiation to human condition attracts more and more attention. The aim of the study [Korotkov, Korotkova , et al 2006] was the detection of responses of people's autonomic nervous system to the mobile phones. 15 practically healthy subjects – volunteers of the age 20-30 years old, all yang women took part in the experiments. People were tested with GDV several times initially and after 5 and 10 minutes speaking on mobile phone kept nearby the ear. The following conclusions were presented by the researchers:

1. Variation of parameters in initial state for all participants during 10 minutes was insignificant, while keeping mobile phone in transmission mode nearby the ear for 10 minutes resulted in statistically significant changes of physiological parameters for most of the tested people. So we may conclude that autonomic nervous system reacted to the influence of the mobile phones of the studied types. Two people had no reaction at all.

2. The level of influence depended on the time of influence: after 5 minutes of using the phone reactions were less significant than after 10 minutes.

3. Reaction to phones of different types was different.

4. From the presented data it is clear that the effect of the mobile phone depends on the time of using, type of the telephone and specific condition of the particular person. In other words, reaction to the mobile phone is very individual and this topic needs attention with elaborated research technique using multiple methodic.

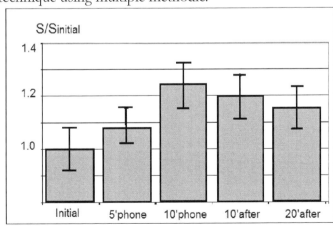

Fig. Relative area of GDV image averaged on 10 fingers for one of the participants. Bars denote standard deviation.

Application of Creams

In the work [Krizhanovski and Lim Kwong Choong 2005] three groups of volunteers with seven people in each group have been investigated to detect their reactions to influence of BAE Synergy Cream, Moisturizing Cream 1 and Whitening Cream 2. Each group was used only one type of cream: Group 1 – BAE Synergy Cream; Group 2 - Moisturizing Cream 1; Group 3 - Whitening Cream 2.

The experiments were done in two stages. At the first stage volunteers were subjected to the POMS test and the GDV-graphy of their fingers at the end of each week during six week.

At the second stage Creams were applied on the subjects' hands each day morning for seven weeks. At the end of each week volunteers also passed the POMS test and the GDV-graphy of their fingers.

As a results of measurements it was shown that the Anxiety GDV parameter have significant decrease after taking BAE Synergy Cream. Significance was shown using Sign and Wilkoxson statistical methods of analysis. After applying Moisturizing Cream 1 and Whitening Cream 2 respectively, the Anxiety factor have a tendency to decrease as well, but the results are not as significant as compared to BAE Synergy Cream. The angle of inclination of average values in case of BAE Synergy Cream was 0.123 compared with 0.045 in case of Moisturizing Cream 1 and 0.089 in case of Whitening Cream 2. Results of POMS test demonstrated that after taking BAE Synergy Cream Tension-Anxiety index of subjects was reducing, while demonstrating no changes in case of other creams. Other POMS parameters did not show any significant changes.

Smelling Essential Oils

The aim of the studies [Prijatkin 2006 and Korotkov, Matravers et al 2008] was to find correlations between objective measurements of the tested individuals reactions to smelling essential oils, subjective evaluation of the odor and the indices of the state of health and psycho-emotional state of the subjects.. The goal was not to evaluate the aroma strength of the oils, but to evaluate their stimulating or calming/ relaxing effects.

32 participants were apparently healthy volunteers 21 ± 2 years old. Before and after the testing participants filled in a special Aveda Essential Oil Evaluation questionnaire. Essential oils were kept in hermetically sealed bottles. All operations with aromas were conducted inside the smell box. Methods of study were Electrocardiography (ECG), EPI /GDV and psychological questionnaires POMS and Aisenk. With EPI the ring (fourth) finger of the left hand was measured at 15-second intervals during a 5-minute baseline/ before smell phase, a 2.5-minute during smell phase at which adaptation to smelling the oil takes place halfway through this phase, and during a 5-minute after smell phase. All 10 fingers were measured with commercial EPI camera before and after smelling.

Peoples' reaction to smelling fragrant essential oils was detected by GDV and HRV methods. Strong correlations between GDV parameters, HRV and psychological indexes were found. Using GDV method one can say, with high probability, what kind of effect an aroma make on particular individual. Experiments showed that perception of different odours depends strongly on personality, and no one can say that concrete odour will always have some definite impact on every individual.

Massage Therapy

Only practically healthy mentally stable people having no allergy reactions were selected for the participation in the experiments [Korotkov, Matravers et al 2008]. More than 100 people participated in experiments, both men and women, age from 21 to 66. Before and after the massage participants filled in a special Mood Mapping Evaluation questionnaire. GDV measurements was administered to the panelists before (baseline) and immediately after massage. Therapists were 6 professional masseurs, 4 men, 2 women, Age 29 ± 6. They were trained for a week in Energy Massage and using essential oils by AVEDA trainer Mark Zelikkofer.

It was shown that for the Energy Massage with essential oils statistically significant changes in GDV indexes were recorded for most of the panellists. For Energy Massage without oils effect was less, but the group effect was statistically significant. For the classical massage the changes was not statistically significant. To make more detailed analysis we may present results as percentage of changes. We calculate the "Parameter of Difference" C in accordance with an equation: $C = (S_{after} - S_{before})/S_{before}*100\%$, where S_{before} and S_{after} - area of an image before and after the massage. Results are presented at Fig. From these graphs we can clearly see the difference in the influence of different types of massage.

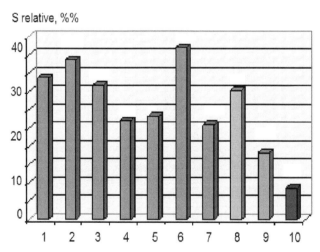

Fig. Increase of GDV area after different types of massage averaged on the group. 1-7 – Chakras 1-7; 8 – Averaged; 9 – Massage without oils; 10 – Classical massage.

Effects of Osteopathy Treatment were studied in the paper of [Korotkov, Shevtsov et al 2012]. 49 apparently healthy adults (20–56 years old) were measured with EPI before, after and 30 min later osteopathy treatment by Dr. Serge Paoletti performed on the whole body. In addition blood pressure, pulse rate, and interference electromyograms were measured. Most of the recipients of these osteopathic treatments experienced increase in fingertip florescence area and average intensity, reduction in stress levels, and improved blood pressure measurements. With all of these parameters simultaneously improving, the patients received a good benefit from these sessions. Especially interesting is the stress level indications measured by the GDV.

Overall the recipients had decreases in their activation coefficient levels. Those who were stressed came into a normal range, and people who were already at normal stress levels stayed there. These results were seen on both the psycho-somatic and physicological, or without and with filter readings. In addition, the levels stayed stable, as shown by the readings done thirty minutes later. Such data can be interpreted as especially meaningful, when even the sympathetic system parameters hold in a relaxed pattern for a length of time.

Dr. Serge Paoletti saw eight patients in each of the eight days, and managed to maintain a stable stress level. He does daily exercises to support his body's natural homeostatic capacities. This is demonstrated by the fact that while his activation coefficient fluctuates, it does so within the range of focused activity, normal levels, to relaxed. Observe that the lower, relaxed levels appear halfway through the day, when he got his one break, for lunch. These numbers show that a doctor does give a significant output of energy to the patients, therefore it is essential for doctors to learn how to care for themselves.

It should be noted that virtually all subjects were in a good mood after treatment. Many of them had pain and muscle tension which disappeared. These changes were reflected in all parameters analyzed, in both psycho-somatic and somatic states. Thus, osteopathic manipulations as administered in these two studies provide good, lasting relaxation. This study also provides the interesting observation that relaxation practices, as done by Dr Paoletti, on a daily basis, enable him to work hard without additional stress.

Influence of textiles

In the work of Ciesielska I.L. [2007, 2008, 2010] to analyze the influence of textiles on Electrophotonic images of human beings in brief contact with those textiles, three different raw materials were chosen: coarse wool – natural, animal fibre, polyacrylonitryl – man-made synthetic polymer fibre and viscose. In all, 20 volunteers (nine men, aged 21-54 years, mean 46 ± 11 years and eleven women, aged 21-57 years, mean 35 ± 12 years) were eligible for the study. A sleeve from the material under study was put on left arm of a person while EPI readings were taken from the ring finger of the right hand.

There were significant statistical differences between parameters of EPI recorded during contact with knitted acrylic fabric and knitted viscose fabric (p=0.0240), knitted acrylic fabric and knitted wool fabric (p=0,0210), knitted acrylic fabric and lack of any fabric (bare arm) (p=0.0080) as well as during contact with knitted wool and viscose fabrics (p=0.4980), viscose and lack of any fabric (p=0.0450) and wool and lack of any fabric (p=0.0340).

– There was no correlation between parameters of EPI in the frame of repetitions of contact with fabrics and without fabric. There are no significant statistical differences between parameters of EPI in the frame of repetition of contact with each textile or without (p=0.5693).

– There were significant statistical differences between the length of radius (p=0.01050) and the coefficient of shape (p=0.0144) in EPI recorded for women and men. Moreover, as regards the mean length of radius, mean brightness, number of fragments of the EPIs recorded during contact of volunteers with knitted fabrics.

– Menstrual cycle of female volunteers; the later the day of the cycle, the higher the value of standard deviation from the mean length of radius and the lower the value of standard deviation of numbers of fragments.

- Gender of volunteers; in EPIs recorded from fingertips of men, the length of isoline is higher than from fingertips of women – it derives from the anatomical differences as usually bigger fingertips are observed in males than females. Age of respondents: the older the person, the higher the value of form coefficient.

The Affect of the Great Pyramid

The current quantitative study used a pre-test–posttest experimental design to measure consciousness fields and the affect of the Great Pyramid on the chakra system [Boulter 2012]. Thirty-nine subjects participated in the study over a three day period from October 9-11, 2010. On the first day of the study, a pre-test was conducted at the Movenpick Hotel in Giza. Special permission was granted by the Supreme Council of Antiquities for private entry into the Great Pyramid for 2 hours beginning at sunrise on 10-10-10. The subjects entered the Great Pyramid and climbed up the Grand Gallery in silence. They entered the Kings Chamber and one by one, they stepped into the granite coffer with 4-inch stone walls and laid down for 2 minutes immediately after being tested on the GDV/EPI device both without filter and with filter. After the 2 hours had passed, all subjects left the Great Pyramid in silence and returned to the bus. The Giza Plateau was then open to the public. On the third day, the posttest was conducted at the Movenpick Hotel. Full data sets for 30 participants were analyzed. Worthy of note, none of the subjects included in the data analysis had been into the Great Pyramid before the study was conducted.

The data showed that mean Chakra values were positive approaching 0.00 balance Inside the Pyramid. Before and After mean values show a greater range with both positive and negative values indicating less balance.

On the Area of Energy Field 3 people demonstrated increase of Energy Field inside the Pyramid compared with Before data, 2 people did not change, and 25 people demonstrated decrease of Energy Field inside the Pyramid compared with Before data.

16 subjects had the strongest energy fields After; 13 subjects were strongest Before; and only 1 subject was strongest Inside the pyramid but only slightly measuring 3.1% greater Area Inside than After.

It seems clear that the pyramid did not affect all subjects in the same way. This stands to reason since, in today's society, initiation and consciousness fields are not well understood and subjects likely did not know how to handle the increased energy. This may be the reason subjects' chakras slipped out of alignment during the study.

The most unexpected finding is that the Energetic Frequency

(measured with Sputnik instrument [Korotkov 2011] outside the Great Pyramid was not only higher, it was also more stable.

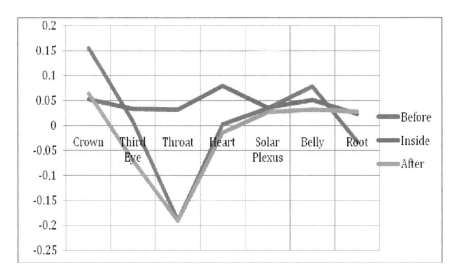

Fig. Plotted means of 7 Chakras for 30 subjects Before, Inside, and After.

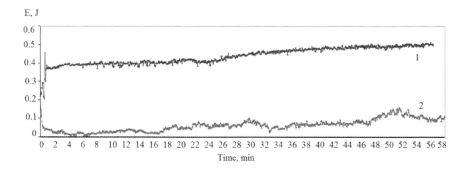

Fig. Energy Frequency Outside (1) and Inside the Great Pyramid over 1 hour.

Psycho-emotional state

The GDV method, can assess general improvement of an emotional condition, removal of emotional and nervous excitation and tension during short-term rehabilitation procedures for more than 700 patients [Sergeev 2004].

Excessively high level of the GDV parameter Entropy can indicate mental disorders, in particular schizophrenia, etc. If the level of GDV-entropy is excessively low, it points to the prospect that this individual may be "running out of options" and he is in danger of "burning out" [O'Keeffe 2006].

Significant relationships between GDV parameters and State anxiety and less significant relationships with Trait anxiety and Neuroticism. Significant relationships are also found for the personality dimensions of Openness and Agreeableness. [Dobson 2007, 2011].

Correlations shown between GDV-gram parameters and the adaptation periods of polar explorers, especially the characteristics of dynamics in the GDV parameter Entropy. The length of adaptation period is quite unique for every participant. Possible adaptation anomalies, such as prolonged adaptation syndrome, can be particularly well disclosed with the described technique of entropy control . By the use of GDV technique it is possible to assess concrete changes in organism systems of a chronic alcoholic person with a high degree of probability. [Om 2004].

In many studies GDV technique was used for detecting effect of spiritual practices, such as prayer, meditation or healing. As an example we present graph from the research conducted in the clinic of psychotherapy and Eastern medicine "Urusvati" (Ukraine, Dnepropetrovsk) Semenihin E.E. and Zheltyakova I.N. [2004]. Prayer was investigated with 11 volunteers, mantra – with 17, meditation – with 15. People have been acquainted only with practice of meditation before, but not with practice of reading aloud prayer or mantra. All people demonstrated increase of their energy parameters after the practice.

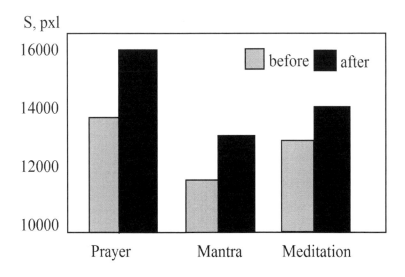

S, pxl

Fig. Changes of EPI indexes after spiritual practice.

A lot of correlations were found between GDV parameters and results of psychological analysis. In the report [Lovygina and Larionov 2005] the following correlations with the Lucher test were found:

	GDV Area	Symmetry
Uneasiness	r = - 0.58-0.66;	r = - 0.83
Activity	r = 0.72-0.76;	r = 0.63
Vegetative tonus	r = 0.47-0.51	r = 0.50

All correlations were statistically significant (p < 0.05).

In the work of Rgeusskaja G.V. and Listopadov U.I. [2009] an idea was proposed that Electrophotonics Technology may be useful in Evaluation of Cognitive Functions.

Bulatova TE, Popova TV and Tarasova MN. [2005] studied peculiarities in GDV-graphy indexes of women under physical and emotional stress influence.

New approach for remote detection of human emotions was offered by Korotkov K, Orlov D and Madappa K. [2009] based on application of a special "Sputnik" sensor.

The aim of the research project in Kaliningrad Federal Institute was evaluation of possible correlations between results of psychological testing and GDV indexes [Vasilenko et al 2012]. 112 yang apparently healthy men mean age 18 +/- 2 years were tested with several questionneries:

Short selection test;

Inner values test after Rokich;

16 factors questioners after Kettel;

Test on multiple parameters of a person.

All-in-all it was 94 psychological parameters which were compared with 144 GDV indexes for every person.

Simple direct correlations did not show significant results. Then equitation of multiple regressions were calculated in Statistica program in the following form:

$$Y = a + b_1 \times X_1 + b_2 \times X_2 + \ldots + b_p \times X_p,$$

Where a – constant; b_1- b_p – regression coefficients; $X_1 – X_p$ – psychological and GDV parameters.

This approach allowed to calculate 63 correlation prognostic models with correlation coefficients 0.91 – 0.99 and statistical value 0,05-0,00001. Models were tested on independent group of people and demonstrated very high prognostic value.

From the success of this work we can draw several conclusions.

1. Further development of prognostic models, both in psychology and in medicine should be based on quite big databases randomized on age and gender.

2. Simple direct correlations may be efficient only in cases of very strong inner bonding, but in most cases we should use multiple regression analysis.

3. We should be careful in applying model generated on particular database to population of different age, gender and even same type of population from different countries.

Sport

43 athletes - members of the juvenile national team of Russia and team of Krasnodar region were evaluated with GDV technology in the training period and results was used for the prediction of the competitive activity [Ozhug, Rusinov 2004]. Significant correlations were found between GDV indexes and psychological parameters of athletes evaluated by several questionnaires: longing to success (r = 0.846); avoiding of failures (r = 0.821); rating in a team (r = 0.812); emotional stability (r = 0.785); self regulation (r = 0.781); anxiety (r = -0.724); tension (r = -0.711). Based on these results the forecast of competition success from made before the competition which proved itself with 95% accuracy.

Big research for several years was conducted in the Dnepropetrovsk institute of physical culture and sport [Rodina et al 2008]. The research has been carried out on the base of the Ukraine national football team and women sitting volleyball team. Strong correlations between psychological parameters of athletes and GDV indexes were found. This research was later developed with the Olympic Ukrainian yachting team during 2009-2010.

Systemic research of GDV applications in sport have been performed in Saint Petersburg Research Institute of Physical Culture and Sport of Russian Ministry of Sport. It was initiated by Professor Pavel Bundzen and after his death led by Professor Konstantin Korotkov and Dr. Anna Korotkova. Many papers have been published in Russian and international per-review journals [Bundzen et al 2000-2005; Korotkova 2006; Drozdovski et al 2012] and a book in Russian "GDV Technique in Sport" (Sport Publishing, Moscow 2007). In the research as examinees took part male and female athletes, champions and participants of Olympic Games and Paralympic Games, the World and European championships, the highly skilled athletes.

A lot of correlations were found between GDV indexes and other parameters both physiological and psychological. After careful analysis of many thousands of studied cases several techniques have been selected for complex evaluation of athletes' level of preparation and competition efficiency:

Heart Rate Variability;
Electrophotonic technique;
Balancing Platform;
Computer processing of video records of athletes performance.

This approach was officially accepted by Russian Ministry of Sport and now is being used in preparation to Olympic and Paralympic Games. In particular, researchers from St Petersburg Institute of Sport helped a lot in preparation to the Paralympic Games 2012 in London working with teams in training camps in preparation period and at the Games. This helped Russian Paralympic Team to get the second place on the medal score after China. Activity of researchers was highly prized by the Ministry of Sport.

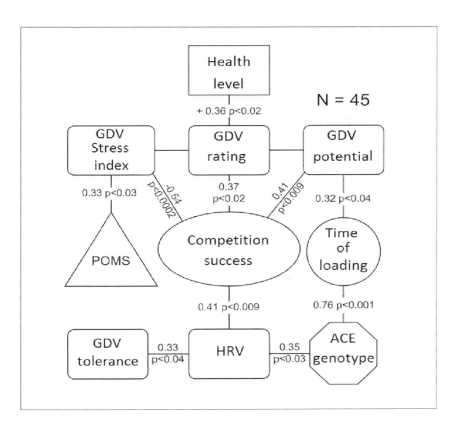

Fig. Correlation factors for top-level athletes. POMS – profile of mood state; HRV – heart rate variability; ACE – angiotenzin converting enzyme [Bundzen et al 2005].

After many years of experience two main EPI/GDV indexes have been selected which was found the most gainful for evaluation athletes' level of preparation: **Energy Potential, calculated from 0 to 100% and Stress (Anxiety) Level, calculated from 0 to 10.** These indexes allow to evaluate the level of individual preparation of a particular athlete, the probability of competition efficiency and rating in a tem. Advantage of this test is its fastness – it takes less than a minute to take a reading and immediately evaluate result. So Russian athletes were evaluated in the morning before the competition and immediately after it was over. Conclusions were very helpful in organizing the training process.

As an example we may present graph of experimental data analysis from [Drozdovski et al 2012]. It shows distribution of parameters between 18 athletes from Russia's Skiing and Biathlon Paralympic Team averaged on the three periods of time: at the training camp, before the World Cup competition and at the moment of World Cup competition. As we see from the graph, all athletes may be divided in three groups: top level athletes (N 12-18) with high EP and low SL mostly by the time of competitions; middle-level athletes (N 4-11) with high EP and moderate SL; and juniors (N 1-3) with low EP and high SL.

Currently, the exact mechanism detailing how a high EP leads to athletic readiness is unclear. However, a theoretical model proposed by the authors postulates that EP may act like a psycho-physiological reservoir for an athlete. The larger the reservoir the more the psycho-physiological resources an individual has access to when energetic resources are demanded, as is the case during athletic competition. If the reservoir is large, then many small, or even few large demands placed upon it will not cause any major depletion. However, if a person begins training with a small energetic reservoir, even tiny demands may prove unbearable and lead to a rapid depletion of EP. For this reason, the hypothesized relative static nature of EP underscores the importance of achieving a high EP during training camp. Once an athlete has their particular EP established they have in essence set their homeostatic EP level. It should be noted that this EP level exhibits relative homeostasis and while this can fluctuate, it generally maintains within a given range for a period of time once it has been set.

Another important aspect of EP is its relationship to stress. In all correlations analyzed, EP was negatively correlated to SL. This was most pronounced for SL at the World Cup. These results suggest that a high EP may serve a protective function against high stress levels. A low-level stress response is the body's normal physiological answer when it is challenged in some way. This adaptation is not only beneficial, but also necessary for the maintenance of health and wellness. When the stress response is disproportionate to the stressor, or the stress response is prolonged in some way, other downstream negative effects can take place. A high EP seems to attenuate the stress response in order to keep SL low and within acceptable levels for health and wellness. However, if an individual has a high SL in conjunction with a low EP, not only is their athletic preparedness compromised, they may actually be in need of medical or psychological intervention.

A second key observation regarding SL is that it exhibits its own degree of homeostasis. Table 3 shows that the SL of an athlete recorded in the training period significantly correlates with the SL both before and at the time of competition. Therefore, the SL's a person records during the training period, will most likely be similar SL's that same person records at different times throughout the training process. Although SL and EP both tend towards homeostasis, it is the belief of the authors that EP serves as the baseline psycho-physiological marker that resists changes in SL, and not the other way around. This is based on the assumption that as athletes trained and competed in different circumstances (training camp, before WC, at WC), their stressors changed as well. If SL were unregulated by some other mechanism, changes in stressors would directly register as changes in SL. It was assumed that as time approached the actual World Cup competition the stressor associated with competing would increase. However, for top-level athletes SL actually decreases as an athlete moved from training camp, to before World Cup, and at the World Cup.

A direct measurement of **Energy Potential and Stress Level** in the fast, non-invasive manner used for this study is a rather new approach developed in recent years in Russia. It has been tested for several years with teams at different athletic levels and sport types. The equipment and procedures have demonstrated high efficiency and reliability. The measuring process takes 1-2 minutes, and can be done practically anywhere. The instruments used may be run either from a power outlet, from a battery or in the latest models from the USB port of computer. In the latest set of EPI programs both EP and SL parameters may be calculated from measuring only two fingers 4R and 4L without filter. This makes the process of measurements very fast and convenient.

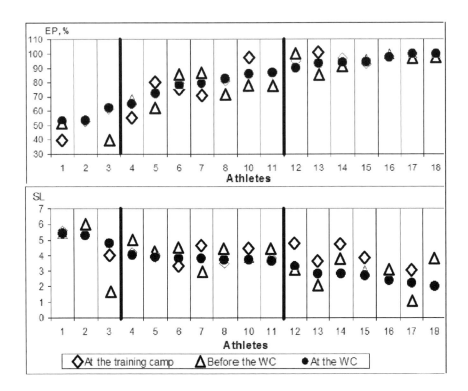

Fig. Energy Potential and Stress Level for individual athletes measured at the different moments: in the training camp; before the competition; at the moment of competitions.

Biological Liquids

The GDV technique enables one to identify specific reaction of antibodies with a complimentary antigen, called agglutination reaction. The technique is based on the registration of dynamics of parameters of blood samples GDV glow in time – from the moment of combination (mixing) of specific components (antigen and antibodies to it) to the moment of completion of their interaction and formation of the so-called immune complexes. As a results of such interaction, physico-chemical characteristics of the investigated material, and consequently, GDV-gram parameters change [Stepanov et al 2004]. Fig. demonstrates the example of GDV blood reaction to different allergens: 1 – initial blood plasma, 2 – blood plasma with egg albumin and 3 – blood plasma with marjoram flower essence. As we see from this picture, there was no reaction to albumin and significant reaction to the flower essence. The technique can be applied for the investigation of nontransparent biological liquids when it is not only difficult, but even impossible to implement the agglutination reaction in its classical form (visual registration of results); for example, study of blood with the purpose of revealing etiology of human allergies.

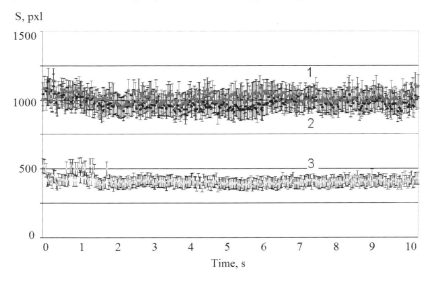

Fig. GDV blood reaction to different allergens: 1 – initial blood plasma, 2 – blood plasma with egg albumin and 3 – blood plasma with marjoram flower essence. Every point is averaged on 10 measurements.

Blinded, randomized assessment of four split samples of homeopathy preparations using GDV technique were conducted in Arizona University [Bell et al 2003]. This study compared the gas discharge visualization (GDV) image patterns generated by 30c potencies (10^{-60}, diluted beyond Avogadro's number and succussed [vigorously shaken] 600 times) of three widely-used homeopathic medicines (Natrum Muriaticum – sodium chloride, Pulsatilla - windflower, Lachesis – Bushmaster snake venom) and two different 20% alcohol-water solvent controls (solvent with untreated lactose pellets, plain solvent alone). GDV form coefficient, area, and brightness were significantly lower for the medicines (Pulsatilla and Lachesis) than the controls at range 3 voltage. However, at range 4 voltage, Natrum Muriaticum and Lachesis had greater form coefficients than did solvent with untreated pellet controls, whereas Pulsatilla had the lowest form coefficient. Repeated imaging of the same drops at range 3 degraded the magnitude of the correlation between the first and subsequent images for the Pulsatilla (plant source) and Lachesis (animal source) more than for Natrum Muriaticum (mineral source) or the solvent controls. Split samples did not show replicable results between bottles of the same test solution. Similar to studies showing that raising pH can release excess heat from ultramolecular doses of homeopathic medicines, the current findings suggest that GDV electrical impulses at certain voltages and over repeated applications may serve as a probe for biophysical properties of homeopathic medicines. Variations in ability of GDV to induce disruption of water cluster patterns, initially formed in accord with the original source molecules of the medicines, may be a mechanism.

Conclusion

Analysis presented in this book was based on 161 papers published from 2000 to 2012 mostly in English (except of some latest papers in Russian). Most of them were presented at the conferences, some published in per-review journals. We did not pretend to cover all works published on the topic (there are more than 200 papers in Russian database only). We did not include publications on water, minerals, plants, etc studies, as well as geo-active zones and quantum Feng Shuai. The aim of this work was to give an overall impression on the scope of Electrophotonic research in medicine and psychology and demonstrate different approaches being used in this field. From the analysis of presented data we can make several conclusions.

$\frac{35}{17}$ A lot of significant correlations between EPI/GDV indexes and psycho-physiological parameters were found. This tells us that Electrophotonic parameters reflect the level of autonomic regulation of the body and its functional reserves. Functional disorders may be or may be not reflected on somatic level of the organism, i.e, organ may have normal appearance on Ultrasound or MRI image, but its functioning may be suppressed. So from classical point of view the organ may be normal, and only functional analysis may reveal the deep reason of the problem, influencing well-being of a person.

$\frac{35}{17}$ Functional level depends both on somatic functioning of the body and on the mental state of a person. Close connection between *soma* and *psyche* allows us to see their mutual influence and distinguish different features using filters and dynamic screening. So Electrophotonic analysis is holistic, integrative approach which takes into consideration both somatic and consciousness activity of a person.

$\frac{35}{17}$ Specially developed models based on particular database of people may have prognostic values for different nosological cases.

$\frac{35}{17}$ At the same time we do not claim Electrophotonic as diagnostic technique.

$\frac{35}{17}$Electrophotonic approach is aimed to generate data on energy potential of different systems and organs of the body and on the level of physiological anxiety of a person. This information, together with the results of other analysis, both conventional and holistic, should allow doctor to develop diagnosis or recommend patient additional specific types of analysis.

$\frac{35}{17}$ Electrophotonic analysis allows spotting the areas of attention, both hipo- and hyper-energy, and, applying filter, define the influence of a psyche component on the particular area. This makes prognostic power of this approach.

$\frac{35}{17}$ Diagnostic Table after Mandel-Korotkov has been proven in many testing, but we need to keep in mind, that sector boundaries are not rigid; they fluctuate and influence each other. We study live active Energy Field which follows circadian rhythms and fluctuate under the influence of an environment. There are many cases when sector analysis is not applicable at all. Detailed discussion of this topic please see in the book [Korotkov K.G. Energy fields Electrophotonic analysis in humans and nature. 2012. 240 p. e-book: Amazon.com] and other editions and translations of this book.

$\frac{35}{17}$ Experienced doctor or practitioner after some training and experience practice can evaluate problems for a patient with probability 80-85%. We know many cases when people were told about hidden problems which were revealed later by detailed analysis.

$\frac{35}{17}$ Reliable information about problems of a patient may be revealed only by following the rules and conditions defined in the first part of this book.

$\frac{35}{17}$ So we see the potential of the EPI analysis as a first level of a diagnostic process, which allows doctor to develop a strategy of the further analyses and treatment. This defines the areas of EPI method application in classical and integrative medicine. The advantages of this approach in that it is non-invasive, fast, reliable and does not depend on the operator. EPI/GDV instruments are ideal for mass-screening of population, in particular in low-developed countries and in cases of field operations: at the battle-fields or in the areas of catastrophes, where it is necessary to test many people in a short time.

$\frac{35}{17}$ We should be very careful in analysis of oncology patients. It is commonly accepted in modern medicine that cancer is not a decease of a particular organ, but system disorder of the whole body. There are many types of cancer and many stages of this process. So oncology patients may have different character of EPI/GDV images, depending on many factors, and we may detect some troubleshooting features only at the images with filter. At the same time we should never tell a patient about our suspicion of oncology process, but only recommend next type of analysis.

$\frac{35}{17}$ Another strong advantage of the EPI technique is its ability to monitor condition of people after different influences. As is shown in many cases presented in this book, EPI technique is very sensitive and allows monitoring practically any type of influence, would it be medical intervention or spiritual practice. This is an ideal instrument for research, as in many cases it allows to follow up reactions of a person, unavailable to other techniques. Many different parameters calculated from the image were being widely used in the research practice and proved the validity of this approach.

$\frac{35}{17}$ EPI instrument is ideal for individual analysis, as people have big variety of reactions to one and the same intervention. So we see strong potential in using EPI instruments as home appliances allowing a person monitor his/her own condition and select the most appropriate types of activity and intervention.

$\frac{35}{17}$ Electrophotonic technique makes a bridge between Western Scientific and Medical approach and Ancient Oriental wisdom. It is based on the notion of Energy Meridians and Energy Fields, it is using the principles of Traditional Chinese Medicine and Aurvedic Medicine and combines them with the power of modern non-linear mathematics. To use this system to full extend one should have at least a basic understanding of these principles.

As we see from the presented data, Electrophotonic analysis finds more and more proponents and a lot of professional benefit from using this approach. Strong scientific basis and a lot of positive responses from all over the world create solid foundation for the wide development of this approach. We are proud that in 17 years of development we had no negative responses from the users of EPI/GDV instruments. For a lot of doctors and practitioners it became an important tool in their everyday practice.

So we are planning a new level of the Electrophotonic development. It will be based on a new set of programs operating through the Internet. New mathematical procedures created by our team allowed speeding up raw data processing thousand times, and modern protocols provide appropriate speed of data exchange. Now there are no need to use different programs for creating information – all is done on the server and user has all the information in several seconds. This allows to simplify the training process and make all upgrades in a most convenient for users way. This software operates on Windows and Mac platforms, as well as with some limitations on different tablet PC. From now on the world of different electronic gadgets is open for Electrophotonic applications.

Next stage – combining EPI instrument with Energy Field correction. In the new programs we generate frequency individual for a person. Based on these frequencies we create music which may be downloaded to the pocket-size electronic device. Person listen this music through the special earphones connected to the device and during 10 min session three times he/she has healing session of Ultra-Hight Frequency (UHF) modulated by the music and generated by special crystals inserted in the earphones.

This way a person has a healing session by frequencies generated from his/her own energy field. After the session it is possible to make a new measurement and generate new corrected music. This is a classical biofeedback regime.

UHF correction is well-known in Russia and for many years is being used in Russian hospitals for stress-reduction and rehabilitation. It is based on many years of research and clinical testing and approved by Russian Ministry of Health.

We hope all these new steps will help further development of Electrophotonic movement in medicine, psychology and other health and well-being applications. Of course this may be done only with the help and support of professionals, so we are waiting for your responses and appreciate and comments and suggestions.

Ekaterina Jakovleva,
Konstantin Korotkov

January 2013

References

1. Abadi M., Streeter T., Ulanowsky D. A Correlation Analysis Between Four Energy Field Scanning Devices And Conscious Perception Of Bodily Issues. In: Proceedings of IX International Scientific Congress on Bioelectrography. St Petersburg 2005:1-3

2. Akhmeteli GG, Baranova TN, Korotkina SA, Pakhomova KS. The experience of using GDV-graphy technique for the determination of rhesus-factor and human blood groups according to ABO system. In: Proceedings of VIII International Scientific Congress on Bioelectrography. St Petersburg 2004:63-66.

3. Akhmeteli GG, Boldyreva US, Komissarov NV, et al. Diagnostics of allergy aetiology using gas-discharge visualization (GDV) technique: Workbook. St Petersburg 2005:39.

4. Alexandrova EV, Zarubina TV, Kovelkova MN, Struchkov PV, Yakovleva EG. GDV Technology – New Step in Diagnostic of the Arterial Hypertension. Vetnik Medicinskich Technologii, 2010 . XVII 1: 122-125 (in Russian)

5. Alexandrova EV, Zarubina TV, Zubkova AV, Kovelkova MN, Struchkov PV, Yakovleva EG. Bioelectrography Approach to analysis of patients with disorders of magisterial head arteries at the extra-cranial level. 2011 XVII 3, 94-96. (in Russian).

6. Alexandrova R. et al. 2001. Energy-informational effects of drugs and acupuncture for bronchial asthma patients. Proceedings of the Saint Petersburg State Medical University. V.8, N 1, pp. 73-78.

7. Alexandrova R. , Fedoseev G., Korotkov K., Philippova N., Zayzev S., Magidov M., Petrovsky I. 2004. Analysis of the Bioelectrograms of Bronchial Asthma Patients. In: Measuring Energy Fields State of the Science. Fair Lawn, NJ, Backbone, , pp

8. Alexandrova RA, Fedoseev BG, Korotkov KG, Philippova NA, Zayzev S, Magidov M, Petrovsky I. Analysis of the bioelectrograms of bronchial asthma patients. In: Proceedings of conference "Measuring the human energy field: State of the science". National Institute of Health. Baltimore, MD, 2003:70-81.

9. Alexandrova RA, Nemtsov VI, Koshechkin DV, Ermolev SU. Analysis of holeodoron treatment effect on cholestasis syndrome patients. In: Proceedings of VII International Scientific Congress on Bioelectrography. St Petersburg 2003:4-6.

119

10.	Alexandrova RA, Trofimov VI, Bobrova EE, Parusova VK. Comparison of dermal allergology test results and changes of GDV bioelectrograms in case of contact with phytocosmetic substance in test tube. In: Proceedings of VII International Scientific Congress on Bioelectrography. St Petersburg 2003:1-4.

11.	Akhmeteli GG, Baranova TN, Korotkina SA, Pakhomova KS. The experience of using GDV-graphy technique for the determination of rhesus-factor and human blood groups according to ABO system. In: Proceedings of VIII International Scientific Congress on Bioelectrography. St Petersburg 2004:63-66.

12.	Akhmeteli GG, Boldyreva US, Komissarov NV, et al. Diagnostics of allergy aetiology using gas-discharge visualization (GDV) technique: Workbook. St Petersburg 2005:39.

13.	**Bell I, Lewis DA, Brooks AJ, et al. Gas Discharge Visualisation Evaluation of Ultramolecular Doses of Homeopathic Medicines Under Blinded, Controlled Conditions. J Altern Complement Med 2003;9;1:25-37.**

14.	Belogorodsky B.A., Sidorov G.A., Yantikova T.A., Yanovskaya E.E. Scenar therapy and application of GDV bioelectrography. In: Proceedings of VIII International Scientific Congress on Bioelectrography. St Petersburg 2004:67-68.

15.	Berne Samuel A. Studies the effect of dolphins on the human biofield using GDV analysis. In: Proceedings of XV International Scientific Congress on Bioelectrography. St Petersburg 2011:24-25.

16.	Bigler C, Weibel FP. Testing agricultural commodities with Gas-Discharge-Visualisation (GDV). In: Proceedings of the International Scientific Conference: Measuring energy fields. Kamnik/Tunjice, Slovenia 2007:93-96.

17.	Bolehan VS, Maltsev OV, Lvov NI, et al. Serosity analysis of influenza and ARD patients by means of Gas Discharge Visualization method. In: Proceedings of X International Scientific Congress on Bioelectrography. St Petersburg 2006:54-55.

18.	Bordes S., Bordes Ch., Korotkov K. Study Of The Human Energy Changes During Caucasus Expedition. In: Proceedings of X International Scientific Congress on Bioelectrography. St Petersburg 2006:3-5.

19.	Bordes S. Sports Nutrition and Altitude (Acclimatization) Interest of Supplementation. In: Proceedings of XV International Scientific Congress on Bioelectrography. St Petersburg 2011: 26-28

20.	Boulter C. The Affect Of The Great Pyramid On The Human Aura And The Chakra System. In: Proceedings of XVI International Scientific Congress on Bioelectrography. St Petersburg 2012: 2-8

21.　　Brezhneva TV, Borovkov EI, Dovgusha VV, et al. Patient state monitoring using GDV method in case of application of autoquantum therapy. In: Proceedings of XI International Scientific Congress on Bioelectrography. St Petersburg 2007:9-12.

22.　　Bikov A.T. and Tchernousova L.D. The Use Of Gas-Discharging Visualization Method (Gdv) In Sanatorium Conditions. In: Proceedings of VIII international Scientific Congress on Bioelectrography. St Petersburg 2003: 36-39.

23.　　Bulanova KJ, Lobanok LM, Ignatenko AO, et al. Gas Discharge Visualization technique in investigation of small ionizing radiation doses affect on human organism. In: Proceedings of X International Scientific Congress on Bioelectrography. St Petersburg 2006:11-12.

24.　　Bulatova TE, Popova TV, Tarasova MN. Peculiarities in GDV-graphy results dynamics of a woman under physical and emotional stress influence. In: Proceedings of IX International Scientific Congress on Bioelectrography. St Petersburg 2005:86-92.

25.　　**Bundzen P., Zagrantsev V., Korotkov K., Leisner P., Unestahl L.-E. Comprehensive Bioelectrographic Analysis of Mechanisms of the Altered State of Consciousness. Human Physiology, 2000, 26, 5, 558-566.**

26.　　**Bundzen P., Korotkov K., Nazarov I., Rogozkin V. Psychophysical and Genetic Determination of Quantum-Field Level of the Organism Functioning. Frontier Perspectives,2002: 11,2,8-14.**

27.　　**Bundzen P., Korotkov K., Unestahl L.-E. Altered States of Consciousness: Review of Experimental Data Obtained with a Multiple Techniques Approach. J of Alternative and Complementary Medicine, 2002, 8 (2), 153-167.**

28.　　Bundzen PV, Korotkov KG, Belobaba O, et al. Correlation between the parameters of induced opto-electron emission (Kirlian effect) and the processes of corticovisceral regulation. In: Proceedings of VII International Scientific Congress on Bioelectrography. St Petersburg 2003:89-91.

29.　　**Bundzen PV, Korotkov KG, Korotkova AK et al. Psychophysiological Correlates of Athletic Success in Athletes Training for the Olympics. Human Physiology. 2005; 31; 3:316–323.**

30.　　Bundzen PV, Korotkov KG, Korotkova AK, et al. Psychophysical potential of sportsmen in Olympic reserve. Collection of guidelines for Russian Olimpic reserve colleges. Orel, 2004:83-103.

31.　　**Bundzen PV, Korotkov KG, Korotkova AK, Priyatkin NS. Psycho-physical prognosis of winnings in sport. J of Medicine and Sport, 2005;2:23-24.**

32.   Bundzen PV, Korotkov KG. Correlation between Psycho-physiological and Genetic Factors for Top-level and Middle-level Athletes in Sports with Physical Endurance. In: Korotkov K, editor. *Measuring Energy Fields*. Fair Lawn: Backbone Publishing, 2004:83-91.

33.   Buyantseva LV, Korotkov KG, Zhegmin Qian, Bascom R, Ponomarenko GN. Gaseous discharge visualization (GDV) bioelectrography in patients with hypertension: pilot study. In: Proceedings of conference "Measuring the human energy field: State of the science". National Institute of Health. Baltimore, MD, 2003:31-54.

34.   Bykov AT, Chernousova LD, Brodnikova NN. Bioelectrography in complex evaluation of adaptation under laser therapy in sanatorium conditions. In: Proceedings of X International Scientific Congress on Bioelectrography. St Petersburg 2006:170-171.

35.   **Ciesielska I.L., Masajtis J. The influence of textiles on corona discharge created around a human fingertip. Fibers & Textiles in Eastern Europe. 2007, 15, 5 – 6, 64 – 65.**

36.   **Ciesielska I.L., Masajtis J. The preliminary studies of influence of garments on human beings' corona discharge. International Journal of Clothing Science and Technology. 2008. 20. N 5. pp 299 – 316**

37.   **Ciesielska I.L. The precursory analysis of the influence of garments on corona discharge created around a human fingertip. Textile research journal, 2010; v. 80: pp. 216 - 225.**

38.   **Ciesielska-Wrobel I.L. Szadkowska I. , Masajtis J., Gosh J.H. Images of corona discharges in patients with cardiovascular diseases as a preliminary analysis for research of the influence of textiles on images of corona discharges in textiles' users. Autex research journal, 2010. v l. 10, n 1, pp 26-30.**

39.   Chesnokova VN, Varentsova IA, Golubina OA. Actual experience with the GDV Bioelectrography in evaluation of a human adaptation to climatographic factors. In: Proceedings of X International Scientific Congress on Bioelectrography. St Petersburg 2006:43-44.

40.   Cioca GH, Giacomoni P, Rein G. A correlation between GDV and heart rate variability measures: a new measure of well being. In: Korotkov K, editor. *Measuring Energy Fields*. Fair Lawn: Backbone Publishing, 2004:59-65.

41.   Cohly H., Kostyuk N., Isokpehi R. and Rajnarayanan R. Bio-electrographic Method for Preventive Health Care. in Proceedings of the 1st IEEE Annual Bioscience and Biotechnology Conference, 2009. 1-4.

42.   Cowan M. and Nunley B. The Effects of Crystal Bowl Toning on the Chakras as Measured by the Gas Discharge Visualization Technique (GDV) and Scores on the Profile of Mood States Scale. Subtle Energies and Energy Medicine. V.16, N 2, pp 37-40, 2005.

43.   Dobson Paul and O'Keffe Elena. Investigations into Stress and it's Management using the Gas Discharge Visualisation Technique. International J of Alternative and Complementary Medicine. June 2000.

44.   Dobson P, O'Keeffe E. Investigation into the GDV Technique and Personality. In: Proceedings of the International Scientific Conference: Measuring energy fields. Kamnik/Tunjice, Slovenia 2007:111-113.

45.   Dobson P, O'Keeffe E. Cognition as a moderator of GDV emission: past research, a current explanation and some ideas for the future. In: Korotkov K.G. Energy fields Electrophotonic analysis in humans and nature. 2012. 240 p. e-book: Amazon.com

46.   Drozdov DA, Shatsillo OI. Analysis of the GDV-bioelectrography images from the positions of vegetology. In: Proceedings of IX International Scientific Congress on Bioelectrography. St Petersburg 2005:3-7.

47.   Drozdovski A., Gromova I., Korotkov K., Shelkov O. Express evaluation of the psycho physiological condition of Paralympic athletes. Open Access Journal of Sports Medicine. 2012 http://www.dovepress.com/article_11692.t14245241

48.   Drozdovski A., Gromova I., Korotkov K. Shelkov O. Psycho-physiological Adaptation of Paralympic Athletes to High Altitudes. Adaptiv Physical Culture. 2012:4,36-38. (in Russian).

49.   Dunlap J.H. Use Of The Gdv In Intercessory Prayer Research: Findings And Considerations. In: Korotkov K (ed): Measuring Energy Fields State of the Science. Fair Lawn, NJ, Backbone, 2004, pp 187–190.

50.   Gagua PO, Giorgobiani LG, Korotkov KG, et al. Gas discharge visualization method in lung carcinoma monitoring during chemotherapy. Georgian Journal of Radiology. Tbilisi 2003;2(15):53.

51.   Gagua PO, Gedevanishvili EG, Kapanidze A, et al. Experimental study of the GDV Technique application in oncology. In: Korotkov KG eds. Measuring Energy Fields: State of the Science. Fair Lawn: Backbone Publishing Co., 2004:43-51.

52. Gagua PO, Gedevanishvili EG, Korotkov KG, et al. Experimental study of the GDV Technique application in oncology. J Izvestia Vuzov – Priborostroenie 2006;49;2:47-50. (in Russian)

53. Garinov G., Korotkov K. Prostate Cancer Groups Statistics Pilot Study. In: Proceedings of XVI International Scientific Congress on Bioelectrography. St Petersburg 2012:56-57.

54. Gedevanishvili EG, Giorgobiani LG, Kapanidze A, et al. Estimation of Radiotherapy effectiveness with Gas Discharge Visualization (GDV). In: Proceedings of VIII International Scientific Congress on Bioelectrography. St Petersburg 2004:98-99.

55. **Gibson s., Williams B. The effect of music and focused meditation on the human energy field as measured by the gas discharge visualization (GDV) technique and profile of mood states. Subtle Energies and Energy Medicine. V.16, N 2, pp 57-60, 2005.**

56. Gimbut V.S. Diagnostic Possibilities Of The Modified GDV Technique In Obstetrics. In: Konstantin G. Korotkov (Ed.). Measuring Energy Fields: Current Research. – Backbone Publishing Co. Fair Lawn, USA, 2004. pp. 65-75.

57. Gimbut VS, Chernositov AV, Kostrikina EV. GDV parameters of woman in phase dynamics of menstrual cycle. In: Proceedings of International Scientific Congresses on Bioelectrography. St Petersburg 2000: 16-19 and 2004:80-82.

58. Gursky VV, Krizhanovsky EV, Korotkina SA, et al. GDV application for diagnostics of patient functional states. In: Proceedings of X International Scientific Congress on Bioelectrography. St Petersburg 2006:180-183.

59. Gursky VV, Krizhanovsky EV, Korotkina SA., Shirokov DM. Characteristics of GDV-grams of patients with various diseases. Proceedings of X International Scientific Congress on Bioelectrography. St Petersburg 2006:177-180.

60. **Hacker GW, Pawlaka E, Pauser G, et al. Biomedical Evidence of Influence of Geopathic Zones on the Human Body: Scientifically Traceable Effects and Ways of Harmonization. Forsch Komplementärmed Klass Naturheilkd,Germany 2005;12:336-342.**

61. **Haydon B, Nunley B. A GDV Comparison of Human Energy Fields Before and After Stimulation of Sheay's Rings of Fire, Earth, Water, Air, Crystal. Subtle Energies and Energy Medicine. V.16, N 2, pp 69-72, 2005.**

62.   Hossu M, Rupert R. Quantum Events of Biophoton Emission Associated with Complementary and Alternative Medicine Therapies. J Altern Complement Med. 2006, 12(2): 119-124.

63.   Ignatiev N.K., Nikolaeva A.A., Gorchakov V.N., Shebolaev I.V., Shumkov O.A., Novgorodtseva G.P., Gorodilova E.V. Bioelectrography as a method of complex diagnosis of functional state of an organism. Proceedings of IV International Scientific Congress on Bioelectrography. St Petersburg 2000:36-37.

64.   Jadad AR, Moore RA, Carroll D, et al. Assessing the quality of reports of randomized clinical trials: Is blinding necessary? Controlled Clin Trials 1996;17:1-12.

65.   Kalashnikova E. 0., Korotkov K. K.,jun Sinkevich V. A., Andreeva A. V., Tomatorin I. V. The Effect Of Music-Therapy On Drug Addicted Juvenile Delinquents. Proceedings of V International Scientific Congress on Bioelectrography. St Petersburg 2001:12

66.   Kartashova N., Pavlov V., Petrickaja E., Zaharov U., Shumskii V. GDV technique in complex treatment of patients with colon cancer. Proceedings of XI International Scientific Congress on Bioelectrography. St Petersburg 2007:157-161.

67.   Kirlian, S.D. and Kirlian, V. Photography and visual observations by means of high-frequency currents. Journal of Scientific and Applied Photography, 1961, V 6, 397-403.

68.   Konikiewicz, L.W. Introduction to Electrography. Leonard's Associates Press. Harrisburg, PA, 1979.

69.   Konikiewicz, L.W and Grif, L.C. Bioelectrography: A new method for detecting cancer and monitoring body physiology. Leonard's Associates Press. Harrisburg, PA, Second Edition,1984.

70.   Kolkin JG, Kolkina VJ. GDV bioelectrography in a modern surgical clinic. In: Proceedings of X International Scientific Congress on Bioelectrography. St Petersburg 2006:183-185.

71.   Korobka IE, Yakovleva EG, Zarubina TV, Korotkov KG. Gender features of vegetative nervous system for healthy people and patients with arterial hypertension. System Analysis in the Biomedical Systems.   2012, 11(3), .572-579. (in Russian)

72.   Korotkov KG (2002) Human Energy Field Study with GDV Bioelectrography, Backbone Pub

73.	Korotkov KG, Polushin US, Levshankov AI, et al. Technical facilities and new quantum biophysics technologies for assessment of human and biological objects state: GDV method. Actual problems in hardware for anesthetization and resuscitation help. St Petersburg 2003:46.

74.	Korotkov K. Experimental Study of Consciousness Mechanisms with the GDV Bioelectrography. In: Science of Whole Person Healing. Volume 2. Rustum Roy (Ed.). New York, Lincoln, Shanghai. 2004. pp. 152-184.

75.	**Korotkov K., Krizhanovsky E., Borisova M., Hayes M., Matravers P., Momoh K.S., Peterson P., Shiozawa K., and Vainshelboim A. The Research of the Time Dynamics of the Gas Discharge Around Drops of Liquids. J of Applied Physics., v. 95, N 7, pp. 3334-3338. 2004.**

76.	**Korotkov K., Williams B., Wisneski L. Biophysical Energy Transfer Mechanisms in Living Systems: The Basis of Life Processes. J of Alternative and Complementary Medicine, 2004, 10, 1, 49-57.**

77.	**Korotkov K, Bundzen P, Bronnikov V, Lognikova L. Bioelectrographic correlates of the direct vision phenomenon. J Altern Complement Med 2005;11;5:885–893.**

78.	**Korotkov KG, Nechaev VA, Petrova EN, et al. Research of GDV fluorescence of human hair. J Izvestia Vuzov – Priborostroenie 2006; 49; 2:51-56. (in Russian).**

79.	Korotkov K., Korotkova A., Petrova E., Serov I., Lukyanov G. Responses Of People To The Mobile Phones And The Influence Of The Protective Devices. . In: Proceedings of XI International Scientific Congress on Bioelectrography. St Petersburg 2007:192-195.

80.	Korotkov K., Matravers P., K. Mommoh, Petrova E., Korotkova A., Shapin A. Correlation Between Objective And Subjective Reactions To Smelling Essential Oils. Influence Of Massage With Essential Oils To Human Energy . In: Proceedings of XII International Scientific Congress on Bioelectrography. St Petersburg 2008:102-108.

81.	**Korotkov K, Orlov D, Madappa K. New Approach for Remote Detection of Human Emotions. Subtle Energies & Energy Medicine • V 19, N 3, pp 1- 15, 2009.**

82.	**Korotkov K.G., Matravers P, Orlov D.V., Williams B.O. Application of Electrophoton Capture (EPC) Analysis Based on Gas Discharge Visualization (GDV) Technique in Medicine: A Systematic Review. The J of Alternative and Complementary Medicine. 2010, 16(1): 13-25.**

83.   Korotkov K., De Vito D., Arem K., Madappa K., Williams B., Wisneski L. Healing Experiments Assessed with Electrophotonic Camera. Subtle Energies & Energy Medicine • V 20, N 3, pp 1- 15, 2010

84.   Korotkov K. Non-local Consciousness Influence to Physical Sensors: Experimental Data. Philosophy Study, 2011, 1, 4, 295-304

85.   Korotkov K, Shevtsov A, Shelkov O, Mohov D, Paoletti S, Mirosnichenko D, Labkovskaya E, Robertson L. Stress Reduction with Osteopathy assessed with GDV Electro-Photonic Imaging: Effects of Osteopathy Treatment. J Alt Compl Med 18, 3: 251-257, 2012.

86.   Korotkova AK. Gas Discharge Visualization bioelectrography method in studies of master-sportsmens psycho-physiology. Abstract of a PhD thesis in psychology. St Petersburg, 2006.

87.   Kostyuk N., Rajnarayanan R. V., Isokpehi R. D., Sims J., Williams B, Korotkov K, Howcroft S, Yeager M, Mann H, Cohly H. H. Bio-electrographic method in detecting heterogeneity and unique features in autism. Int. J. Environ. Res. Public Health 2009, 6

88.   Kostyuk N., Rajnarayanan R. V., Isokpehi R. D., Cohly H. H., "Autism from a biometric perspective," International Journal of Environmental Research and Public Health, vol. 7, no. 5, pp. 1984–1995, 2010.

89.   Kostyuk N., Meghanathan N., Isokpehi R., Cohly H. H. P., "Clustering model to identify biological signatures for English language anxiety," in Proceedings of the 2nd Annual ORNL Biomedical Science and Engineering Conference (BSEC '10), Oakridge, Tenn, USA, May 2010.

90.   Krashenuk AI, et al. Wave effects of medical leeches. In: Korotkov K, editor. *Measuring Energy Fields*. Fair Lawn: Backbone Publishing, 2004:95-103.

91.   Krashenuk AI, Danilov AD, Korotkov KG. Investigation of system optimization of vegetative nervous system work under hirudotherapy impact as a result of comparative analysis of GDV signal and cardiorythm nonlinear analysis. In: Proceedings of X International Scientific Congress on Bioelectrography. St Petersburg 2006:31-35.

92.   Krizhanovsky EV, Borisova MV, Lim KC, Chan TS. Estimation of mineral water's influence on the human body state by means of GDV bioelectrography. J Izvestia Vuzov – Priborostroenie 2006;49;2:62-66.(in Russian)

93.   Krizhanovsky E., Lim Kwong Choong The Study Of Influence Of Bae Synergy Cream On Human Psycoemotional State By Gdv-Graphy And Poms Test. In: Proceedings of IX International Scientific Congress on Bioelectrography. St Petersburg 2005:21-26.

94.   Kupeev VG. Zagumennikov S.U. Capabilities of GDV method in analysis of different treatment-and-reducing measures effectiveness in case of different chronic pathologies of internals. In: Proceedings of X International Scientific Congress on Bioelectrography. St Petersburg 2006:135-138.

95.   Lovygina ON., Larionov S.A. Correlation Of Metrics Gdv-Bioelectrography And Lusher's Test. . In: Proceedings of IX International Scientific Congress on Bioelectrography. St Petersburg 2005:19-21.

96.   Lovygina ON. The method of gas discharge visualization within the system of assessment of vegetative functions in sportsmen's organisms. In: Proceedings of IX International Scientific Congress on Bioelectrography. St Petersburg 2005:21-22.

97.   Lyapko N.G., Lutskyy I.S., Arshinova-Lyapko Yu.N., Levchenko A.Yu. Gas-Discharge Visualization In Effectiveness Evaluation Of Various Metals Multi-Needle Application Therapy With Patients Suffering From Wound Dystrophy Of Spinal Cord. In: Proceedings of XI International Scientific Congress on Bioelectrography. St Petersburg 2007:165-167.

98.   Mamedov UE, Zverev VA. GDV-graphy as a method of express diagnostics and screening control of psychosomatic pathology in contemporary medicine practice. In: Proceedings of IX International Scientific Congress on Bioelectrography. St Petersburg 2005:110-111.

99.   Mamedov UE. Diagnostic potential of GDV-graphy in eduction of musculoskeletal and bronchopulmonary system's pathologies. In: Proceedings of X International Scientific Congress on Bioelectrography. St Petersburg 2006:38-39.

100.   Martin E G. Influencia del Biocom LUX (luz pulsada) en tratamientos terapéuticos en seres humanos. In: Proceedings of XV International Scientific Congress on Bioelectrography. St Petersburg 2011:45-48

101.   Mercier Béatrice, Prost Josiane GDV Use For The Evaluation Of Bol D'air Jacquier® Breathing Session On Human Energy Fields. In: Proceedings of XV International Scientific Congress on Bioelectrography. St Petersburg 2011:49-52

102.		Moss, T. and Johnson, K., Bioplasma of Corona Discharge, in Krippner, S. and Rubin, D. Galaxies of Life: The Human Aura in Acupuncture and Kirlian Photography, Gordon and Breach Science Publishers, Inc, 1973.

103.		O'Keeffe E. The GDV technique as an aide to stress assessment and its potential application in recruitment and selection of individuals suited to positions associated with high level of stress. In: Proceedings of X International Scientific Congress on Bioelectrography. St Petersburg 2006:202-204.

104. Olalde J. Teoría Unificada de Systemics y mas de 500 fórmulas terapéuticas. 2003; Venezuela. Editorial Adaptógenos Internacionales C.A.

105.		Olalde JA, Magarici M, Amendola F, del Castillo O. Correlation between Electrophoton s values and diabetic foot amputation risk. In: Proceedings of Conference: Neurobiotelekom. St Petersburg 2004:54-58.

106.		Om SN, Gursky VV. Research of the characteristics of adaptation syndrome in Antarctica by means of gas discharge visualization technique. In: Proceedings of VIII International Scientific Congress on Bioelectrography. St Petersburg 2004:15-21.

107.		Om SN. Chronic alcoholism diagnosis by means of Gas Discharge Visualization technique. In: Proceedings of VIII International Scientific Congress on Bioelectrography. St Petersburg 2004:92-96.

108.		Ozhug N.N., Rusinov G.R. Using the method of GDV - bioelectrography in the estimation of the competitive reliability of the athletes-shooters from Russian juvenile national team. Proceedings of VIII International Scientific Congress on Bioelectrography. St Petersburg 2004:97-103.

109.		Papuga P. Methodological difficulties in GDV evaluation in patients with hyperthyroidism. In: Proceedings of the International Scientific Conference: Measuring energy fields. Kamnik/Tunjice, Slovenia 2007:113-116.

110.		Pavlov VS, Petritskaya EN, Abaeva LF. GDV method implementation in studies of serum luminescence in cases of different pathologies. In: Proceedings of XI International Scientific Congress on Bioelectrography. St Petersburg 2007:21-22.

111.		**Pehek, J.O., Kyler, H.J., Faust, D.L. Image modulation in corona discharge photography. Science, Vol 194, 263-270, 1976.**

112.		Petritskaya EN, Pavlov VS, Kartashova NV, et al. Evaluation of bioresonance therapy influence on human organism using GDV method. In: Proceedings of X International Scientific Congress on Bioelectrography. St Petersburg 2006:39-40.

113. Pitirimova TN, Cheryakova IS, Pizhova EG. Application of GDV method in alternative medicine. In: Proceedings of X International Scientific Congress on Bioelectrography. St Petersburg 2006:40-42.

114. Polushin US, Korotkov KG, Strukov EU, Shirokov DM. First experience of using GDV method in anasthetization and resuscitation. In: Proceedings of VII International Scientific Congress on Bioelectrography. St Petersburg 2003:13-14.

115. Polushin J, Strukov E.U., Levshankov A, Shirokov D, Korotkov K. Opportunities Of Gas Discharge Visualization Technique In The Estimation Of Functional State Of The Organism In Monitoring Of Patients State After Abdominal Surgery In Perioperative Period With The GDV Camera. In: Konstantin G. Korotkov (Ed.). Measuring Energy Fields: Current Research. – Backbone Publishing Co. Fair Lawn, USA, 2004. pp. 51-58.

116. **Polushin J, Levshankov A, Shirokov D, Korotkov K. Monitoring Energy Levels during treatment with GDV Technique. J of Science of Healing Outcome.. 2:5. 5-15, 2009.**

117. Popova TV, Bulatova TE, Tarasova MN, et al. Personality-oriented correction approach to a student health improvement problem. In: Proceedings of X International Scientific Congress on Bioelectrography. St Petersburg 2006:146-150.

118. **Priyatkin NS, Korotkov KG, Kuzemkin VA, et al. GDV bioelectrography in research of influence of odorous substances on psycho-physiological state of man. J Izvestia Vuzov – Priborostroenie 2006;49;2:37-43. (in Russian)**

119. Rabe L. Evaluation Of Training Sessions For The Emf Balancing Technique Using The Gdv/Epi Measurement Technology. In: Proceedings of XIII International Scientific Congress on Bioelectrography. St Petersburg 2009:139-141

120. Rizzo-Roberts NR, Shealy N, Tiller W. Are there electrical devices that can measure the body's energy state change to an acupuncture treatment. In: Korotkov K, editor. *Measuring Energy Fields*. Fair Lawn: Backbone Publishing, 2004:31-39.

121. **Rgeusskaja G.V., Listopadov U.I. Medical Technology of Electrophotonics – Gas Discharge Visualization - in Evaluation of Cognitive Functions. J of Science of Healing Outcome..2, 5,15-17, 2009.**

122. Rodina J. D., Ovcharenko S.V., Malojvan J.V. Psychological Aspects of Disabled Sportsmen Training And The Usage of Gas Discharge Visualization Technique. In: Proceedings of XIII International Scientific Congress on Bioelectrography. St Petersburg 2009:138-139.

123. Rubik B. Scientific Analysis of the Human Aura. In: In Korotkov K (ed): Measuring Energy Fields State of the Science. Fair Lawn, NJ, Backbone, 2004, pp 157–170.

124. **Rubik B., Brooks A. Digital High-Voltage Electrophotographic Measures of the Fingertips of Subjects Pre and Post-Qigong. Evidence Based Integrative Medicine. 2 (4), 245-242, 2005.**

125. **Russo M. Russo M, Choudhri AF, Whitworth G, Weinberg AD, Bickel W, and Oz MC. Quantitative analysis of reproducible changes in high-voltage electrophotography. J of Alternative and Complementary Medicine 2001, 7, 6, 617-629.**

126. Saeidov W. Living water from Tunjice and its properties. In: Proceedings of the International Scientific Conference: Measuring energy fields. Kamnik/Tunjice, Slovenia 2007:38-39.

127. Saeidov W. The Possibility Of Using Electrophotonics In The Early Diagnosis Of Polyps And Colon Cancer. In: Proceedings of XIV International Scientific Congress on Bioelectrography. St Petersburg 2010:22-23.

128. Savitskaja G. 2001. Inflammatory process in bronchus and GDV-graphy. Vestnik of the North-West Medical Technical Academy. St. Petersburg, pp. 59-65.

129. Semenihin E.E., Zheltyakova I.N. Possibilities of Bioeletctrographics for investigation of energetic nteraction in the system "Human being – Universe". In: Proceedings of VIII International Scientific Congress on Bioelectrography. St Petersburg 2004:78-81.

130. Semenikhin E.E., Zeltyakova I.N., Kozlov A.V, Kozlova N.V. Assessment Of Individual Influence Of The Music Therapy By Means Of GDV Technique. In: Proceedings of XV International Scientific Congress on Bioelectrography. St Petersburg 2011:56-61.

131. **Senkin VV, Ushakov IB, Bubeev UA, Stepanov VK. GDV bioelectrography method in air and space medicine. J Izvestia Vuzov – Priborostroenie 2006;49;2:57-61.(in Russian)**

132. Senkin VV, Ushakov IB, Bubeev UA. Bioelectrographic criteria of overload tolerance of summer pilot team in centrifuge expert test. In: Proceedings of Conference: Neurobiotelekom. St Petersburg 2004:69-70.

133. Senkin VV. Peculiarities of bioelectrographic diagnosis as a reflection of oriental medicine syndrome presence. In: Proceedings of X International Scientific Congress on Bioelectrography. St Petersburg 2006:42-43.

134.   Sergeev SS, Pisareva SA. The use of gas-discharging visualization method (GDV) for monitoring a condition of the personnel at short-term rehabilitation. In: Proceedings of VIII International Scientific Congress on Bioelectrography. St Petersburg 2004:128-129.

135.   Shabaev VP, Kolpakov NV, Muminov TA, et al. Results and future prospects of GDV-graphy application for differentional diagnostics and monitoring of the treatment of lungs tuberculosis and profound of mycosis fungoides – zaaminelles. In: Proceedings of VIII International Scientific Congress on Bioelectrography. St Petersburg 2004:117-118.

136.   Sharkov V., Bagirov E. Complex experiments in the process of healing sessions. In: Proceedings of XV International Scientific Congress on Bioelectrography. St Petersburg 2011:54-56

137.   Sharma B. Biophoton Emission At Fingertips In Diabetes Using Gas Dicharge Visualization. In: Proceedings of XV International Scientific Congress on Bioelectrography. St Petersburg 2012:64-67

138.   Stepanov A, Sviridov L, Korotkina SA, Achmeteli GG, Krizhanovsky EV. Application of the GDV-graphy technique for the estimation of antigen-antibody reaction. In: Korotkov K, editor. *Measuring Energy Fields.* Fair Lawn: Backbone Publishing, 2004:39-43.

139.   Stockley MA, Spiwak AJ. Blood pressure measurement. The Gale Encyclopedia of Surgery and Medical Tests. Ed. Brigham Narins. 2nd ed. Detroit: Gale, 2009. 4 vols.

140.   Strukov EU. Facilities of Gas Discharge Visualization method for assessment of functional state of organism in preoperational period. Abstract of a medical doctoral candidate's thesis. St Petersburg, Military Medical Academy, 2003.(in Russian)

141.   Strukov EU. Tuzhikova N.V. Monitoring of GDV Parameters To Predict The Development of Postoperative Delirium. . In: Proceedings of XIV International Scientific Congress on Bioelectrography. St Petersburg 2010:24-26.

142.   Telesheva T.Yu., Gursky V.V., Kryzhanovsky E.V. Statistical Model Of The Patient Diagnosis Based On Parameters Of Gdv-Grams. In: Proceedings of IX International Scientific Congress on Bioelectrography. St Petersburg 2005:105-106.

143.   Tereshkin S., Korotkov K., Korotkova A. Change Of Chakra Energy In The Process Of G Gom Tum-Mo Yoga Practice. In: Proceedings of X International Scientific Congress on Bioelectrography. St Petersburg 2006:145-146.

144. Tumanova AL. Comparative analysis of GDV bioelectrography results in clinical practice. In: Proceedings of XI International Scientific Congress on Bioelectrography. St Petersburg 2007:26-27.

145. Tumanova AL. Rehabilitation of eye diseases in sanatoria and health resorts practice. In: Proceedings of XI International Scientific Congress on Bioelectrography. St Petersburg 2007:27-29.

146. Vainshelboim AL, Hayes MT, Korotkov K, Momoh KS. GDV Technology Applications for Cosmetic Sciences. IEEE 18th Symposium on Computer-Based Medical Systems (CBMS). Dublin, Ireland June 2005.

147. **Vainshelboim AL, Hayes MT, Momoh KS. Bioelectrographic testing of mineral samples: A comparison of techniques. J Altern Complement Med 2005;11;2:299-304.**

148. **Vepkhvadze R, Gagua R, Korotkov KG, et al. GDV in monitoring of lung cancer patient condition during surgical treatment. J Georgian oncology. Tbilisi 2003; 1(4):60.**

149. Vasilenko SV, Kozik SV, Karnatovskaya NI. Evaluation of Psychological State by Gas Discharge Visualization. Proceedings of the International Conference "Ecology and Health" Kaliningrad, 2012:69-71.

150. Vilner N.S., Spizina E.A. Investigation Of Bronchial Asthma Patients Using Gas Discharge Visualization Technique. In: Proceedings of VI International Scientific Congress on Bioelectrography. St Petersburg 2002:54-58.

151. Voeikov VL, Volkov AV, Senkin VV, et al. Comparative characteristics of diagnostic criteria complex and assessment of effectiveness of bioadaptive method "biophotonic" on the functional state of the body. In: Proceedings of VIII International Scientific Congress on Bioelectrography. St Petersburg 2004:77-80.

152. Volkov AV, Telesheva TU, Gursky VV, Krizhanovsky EV. Influence of the hydrogen peroxide treatment procedure on the GDV-parameters of patients. In: Proceedings of IX International Scientific Congress on Bioelectrography. St Petersburg 2005:28-33.

153. Volkov AV, Telesheva TU, Gursky VV, Krizhanovsky EV. Statistical model of patient diagnosis based on different parameters of GDV-grams. In: Proceedings of IX International Scientific Congress on Bioelectrography. St Petersburg 2005:27-28.

154.   Volkov AV, Telesheva TU, Kondakov SE. Application of modified GDV Bioelectrography method in determination of individual sensitivity to foodstuffs by example of serum study. In: Proceedings of X International Scientific Congress on Bioelectrography. St Petersburg 2006:16-18.

155.   Volkov AV, Telesheva TU. Some phenomenology aspects of induced by GDV method bioelectrographic activity of human. In: Proceedings of X International Scientific Congress on Bioelectrography. St Petersburg 2006:14-16.

156.   Volkov AV, Hunderyakova NV, Telesheva TU, Kondrashiva MN. Characteristics and state of organism correlation investigation by means of GDV method and by activity of succinate dehydrogenase in lymphocytes. In: Proceedings of XI International Scientific Congress on Bioelectrography. St Petersburg 2007:12-15.

157.   Volkov A.V., Egorov V.V., Telesheva T.Yu. Field, Gdv And Haemodiagnostics Of Food Products. In: Proceedings of XIV International Scientific Congress on Bioelectrography. St Petersburg 2010:15-17.

158.   Williams B. How does gas discharge visualization technique assess a body? Emerging models of energy and control in biophysics and physiology. In: Proceedings of X International Scientific Congress on Bioelectrography. St Petersburg 2006:211-214.

159.   Yakovlev VP, Zinatulin SN, Zhdanov AN. Investigation of respiratory maneuvers influence on autonomic nervous system state using Gas Discharge Visualization technique. In: Proceedings of X International Scientific Congress on Bioelectrography. St Petersburg 2006:44-45.

160.   Yakovleva EG, Struchkov PV, Zarubina TV, et al. Evaluation of GDV technique diagnostic possibilities in examination of the patients afflicted with arterial hypertension. In: Proceedings of X International Scientific Congress on Bioelectrography. St Petersburg 2006:216-218.

161.   Yakovleva EG, Struchkov PV, Zarubina TV, Kondratova E.U. Evaluation Of Gdv Diagnostic Potential For Detection Of Patients With Main Arterial Involvement On Extracranial Level And Left Ventricular Hypertrophy. In: Proceedings of XII International Scientific Congress on Bioelectrography. St Petersburg 2008:111-113

Made in the USA
San Bernardino, CA
27 March 2013